Herbs for Life

A Reference for the Modern Herbalist

From the Journals of

K.J. Daoud

Captiva Press

Captiva Press
Placida Publishing, LLC

Placida Publishing, LLC
www.placidapublishing.com

Publisher's Disclaimer

The author of this book is not a medical professional, and the information in this book is in no way intended to replace proper medical care and/or treatment. Seek the advice of a qualified physician and consult with your pharmacist before undertaking any regimen. (Or veterinarian if wanting to apply the information to treating an animal.) While care was taken to insure the accuracy of the information in this book, the publisher and author assume no liability for the direct or indirect use, misuse, or results from the utilization of information in this book. Opinions of uses of plants and herbals in this book are those of the author.

The information in this book is neither endorsed nor verified by the publisher, is not guaranteed to treat or cure any condition or ailment, and is for educational, research, and/or entertainment purposes only.

Use and/or misuse of some of the plants and herbs listed in this book is illegal in some locales. It is the responsibility of the reader to familiarize themselves with local laws and restrictions before undertaking any regimen using the contents listed within.

Use at your own risk after taking all due precautions.

Placida Publishing, LLC.
Imprint: Captiva Press
www.captivapress.com

Herbs for Life

Ebook ISBN: 978-1-936356-18-8
Print ISBN: 978-1-936356-17-1

First Printing: June 2011

This book contains information regarding herbs, plants, and other botanicals. The publisher and author are not liable for any direct or indirect results from the use or misuse of the information in this book. Consult with your physician and pharmacist before using any information in this book. Use at your own risk.

Any medications or trademarked/patented substances mentioned in this book are the properties of the respective owners. They are included for reference only and are in no way an endorsement of the book by said companies.

For errata, visit our website at http://captivapress.com

Placida Publishing, LLC
http://placidapublishing.com

Dedication

I dedicate this book to all of the herbalists and naturalists of the world who use herbalism to help others, to heal the sick and to grow closer to our earth in all its wonder.

Special thanks to those who have supported me in my quest to learn about herbal medicine, tutored me in the workings of the herbs, and convinced me to publish my journals as a book: Jim S., Wilma T. and the members of Annwn.

To my husband, George, for his support throughout the process of all of the re-writes, as well as hair pulling, red-eyed sleepless nights of research and a couple of lost vacations due to me writing constantly. This book was long in the making and two incredible men, George and Brent, helped me with research, travel and the testing of usages of herbs for this book, each putting in several years of help. (Not to mention being my guinea pigs for some of the recipes.) I am grateful to them both.

To my mother, Sharon, for believing in me and showing me the kind of unconditional love and support only a mother (and friend) possesses.

I also thank my editor, Char, for all her hard work and great job editing this book. In addition, I thank everyone who worked so hard on getting this book out—Steph, Les, and Bruce. They all spent many sleepless nights working on this. Thank you all!

Last and never least, to Mother Nature, without whom this book would not exist.

Table of Contents

Part One

Herbs Listed Alphabetically

Foreword

This book is not intended to replace the advice and care of a qualified physician and is merely a guide for seasoned herbalists who already have a working knowledge and respect of the herbs. This is not intended for beginners or those who would use herbs in a dangerous or abusive manner. Herbs are medicine and can harm people and animals. Use caution when purchasing and using herbs. Also use common sense and gather as much information as possible on each herb before using them on yourself or anyone else. This book is not all-inclusive nor does it claim to cure any health problems, make diagnoses, or recommendations for cures or health issues.

The entries in this book are gathered from both old and new resources and reflect both old and new thoughts on using the herbs listed. The herbs are not reviewed in depth in this book and it is recommended that the reader already have an extensive prior working knowledge of herbal medicine before using this reference.

Various poisons have been listed to show why they should be avoided, along with possible remedies, if any. Use of these particular herbs is not recommended and, in many locations, is illegal. Use of this information to knowingly harm yourself, other persons, or animals may be punishable by law. The author and the publisher accept no responsibility for the misuse of this information.

Dosages listed are average, common dosages for healthy adults of an average weight. They must be adjusted properly for age, weight and circumstance. Dosages are based on use of the whole herb and not extracts or standardizations, unless otherwise noted.

Habitats listed are both indigenous and cultivated in the spirit of listing where the herbs may be found today.

Information about each herb is listed in the order of warnings, indications, and then any other helpful information, such as recipes.

Agrimony

Agrimonia Eupatoria
Rose Family
Part Used: Herb, harvested after flower
Habitat: England, throughout as a weed; southern Scotland.

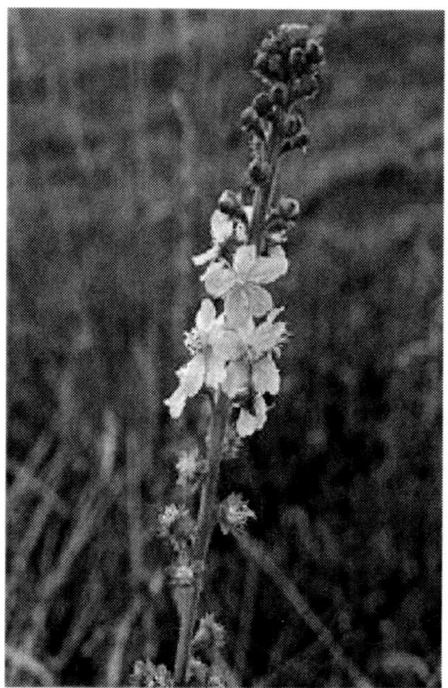

Also known as: Dog Burr; Church Steeples; Cockeburr; Garclive; Liverwort; Philanthropos; Sticklewort; Stickwort

Dosage: 30 - 60 grains

- Do not take with pectin fibers (apples, prunes, etc.) - may cause intestinal blockage
- May aggravate constipation

Primary Uses:
Antibacterial (expels staphylococcus, E. coli, typhoid, dysentery)
Astringent
Bedwetting
Bladder, stones
Cirrhosis
Cough
Diarrhea
Digestion - promotes
Diuretic
Fever
Gout
Healing by stimulating cell growth
Jaundice - tea with honey 3x a day
Kidneys, stones
Liver problems, all
Parasites - expels

Secondary Uses:
Arthritis
Blood clotting - promotes
Cancer, leukemia, ovarian, breast - helps produce "B" cells
Colitis
Detox
Diabetes - lowers sugars in blood
Typhoid Fever
Ulcers, peptic

External Uses:
Antibacterial
Athlete's foot
Bleeding
Bruises
Inflammation, throat - gargle
Pimples
Skin, itchy
Snake bite
Sores
Sprains
Wounds - heals

- Safe for children.

Alfalfa

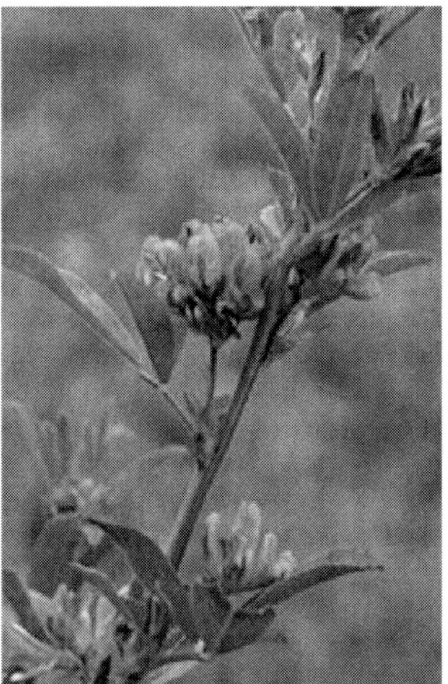

Medicago sativa
Legume Family
Part Used: Whole herb in flower
Habitat: Worldwide, grasslands.

Also known as: Buffalo Herb; Cultivated Lucern; Lucerne; Purple Medicle

Dosage: 60 grains

- May aggravate lupus and other autoimmune disorders.
- **Do not use during pregnancy**.
- Do not use with Premenstrual Syndrome.
- Do not use in presence of a fever.
- Never use unsprouted seeds. They contain high levels of the toxic amino acid canavanine.
- Contains vitamin K, a blood clotter.

Primary Uses:
Arthritis
Colon disorders
Constipation
Detox
Digestive disorders
Diuretic
Immune system - stimulates
Joints, tissue
Liver disorders
Nosebleed - clots blood
Nutritive
Rheumatism
Ulcers, peptic, intestinal

Secondary Uses:
Anti-fungal
Appetite stimulant - tea
Bladder inflammation
Diabetes with manganese
Endometriosis
Inflammation, bladder
Menopause, symptoms
Nausea
Osteoporosis
Pituitary gland function - promotes
Urinary tract infections

Other Possible Uses:
Alcoholism - helps stop
Anemia
Asthma
Cancer - counteract effects of chemotherapy
Cystitis
Dropsy - relieves
Hemorrhoids
High blood pressure
High cholesterol
Hormonal balance - helps
Narcotic addiction - stops
Nursing - good for mothers
Pregnancy - good for
Weight, increases - infusion

External Uses:
Athlete's foot
Bleeding gums
Breath odor
Burns
Decayed teeth - helps rebuild
Skin disorders
Increases production of white blood cells.
Increases cow's milk.

- Infusion: 1 ounce to 1 pint in 1 cupful doses.

Aloe Vera

Aloe barbadenis
Lily Family
Part Used: Leaves
Habitat: East and South Africa; Mediterranean; tropical countries; West Indies.

Also known as: Cape Aloe

Dosage: 1 - 5 grains or 1 - 3 tbsp. Drink between meals only.

- **Do not use during pregnancy - triggers uterine contractions.**
- Do not use during menstruation or if you normally have excessive menstrual flow.
- Do not use with heart medications - produces dangerous heart rhythm abnormalities.
- **Do not use while nursing.**
- Do not use in presence of Crohn's disease, ulcerative colitis or appendicitis.
- If rash develops, discontinue use.
- Do not take with oral contraceptives.
- May increase risk of toxic calcium buildup if taken with calcium carbonate.
- Affects absorption speed of prescription drugs.
- May deplete potassium.
- Abuse may damage colon.

Primary Uses:
Constipation
Laxative
Stimulant
Stomach irritation
Worms

Secondary Uses:
AIDS
Anti-inflammatory
Blood sugar - normalizes
Cancer, all
Diabetes (without weight gain) - leaves
Hangover
HIV
Kidney stones - prevents
Ulcers, peptic

External Uses:
Anesthetic - mild
Antibacterial
Anti-fungal
Anti-inflammatory
Antiviral
Bug bites
Eczema
Frostbite
Hemorrhoids
Itching
Pain
Poison ivy
Psoriasis
Radiation exposure
Scarring - prevents
Skin disorders
Surgical incisions
Swelling
Wounds - accelerates healing
Wrinkles

- When buying aloe vera juice, try to get it without added sugars, etc. The additives may make it taste better, but generally defeat the purpose of drinking the juice in the first place.
- Make sure any gel is not made from aloe latex. If cramps or diarrhea develop, it could be due to aloe latex. Throw out and obtain a new source.
- Leaves may be removed without damage to the plant once they are one inch long.

Angelica

Angelica Archangelica
Parsley Family
Parts Used: Roots, Leaves, Seeds
Habitat: Iceland; Scotland; Syria native; cold, wet northern areas.

Also known as: Angel Root; Archangel; Garden Angelica; Wild Parsnip

Dosage: 10 - 30 grains

- Do not use in presence of diabetes - causes an increase of sugar in urine.
- **Do not use during pregnancy**.
- Large doses may affect blood pressure, heart action and respiration.
- Increases sensitivity to sun (photosensitivity).
- Potentially toxic.

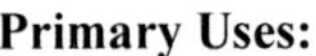

Primary Uses:
Bronchitis, chronic
Colds - hot tea
Colic
Coughs
Emmenagogue, strong - tea
Expectorant - also facilitates other expectorants
Gas - infusion, very fast and gentle for children
Heartburn
Indigestion
Phlegm buildup
Stimulant - aromatic
Stomachic

Secondary Uses:
Anemia, cold hands and feet
Angina
Antiseptic, internal
Bladder infection
Circulation - promotes to the extremities
Diuretic - mild
Fever
High blood pressure
Perspiration - produces
Pleurisy - tonic, infusion
Spasms, stomach & bowels
Urinary organ disease
Warming
Other Possible Uses
Afterbirth - expels, tea
Alcohol - stops cravings
Bites
Digestion problems
Fasting - eat 30 grains powder to guard against
infection
Gout - dried stem juice
Menstrual cramps
Rheumatism - dried stem juice
Typhoid

External Uses:
Aromatic
Baths
Eyes - poultice
Gout - compress
Lice - kills and helps itching
Lung & chest disease - poultice of fresh leaves
Perfume
Rheumatism

- Use freshly cut stalks in the garden to trap earwigs.
- Infusion: 1 pint boiling water, poured over 1ounce herb. Take 2 tbls. 3 times a day.
- Drink: 1 quart boiling water poured over 6 ounce cut up root, 4 ounces honey, juice of 2 lemons and ½ cup brandy. Infuse for ½ hour.

Anise

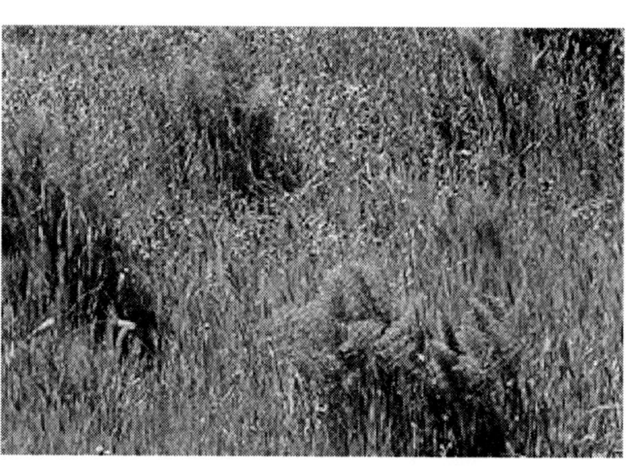

Pimpinella anisum
Parsley Family
Part Used: Seeds
Habitat: Asia Minor; central Europe; Crete; Egypt; Greece.

Also known as: Anise Cultive; Aniseed; Anneys; Pimpinel Seed; Sweet Anise; Sweet Cumin

Dosage: 10 - 30 grains or 4 - 20 drops essential oil

- Large doses are narcotic and slow down circulation.
- **Do not take during pregnancy until ready to deliver - stimulates childbirth.**

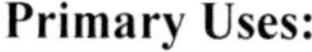

Primary Uses:
Bronchitis - oil mixed with wine
Chest complaints, all
Colds
Coughs, hard and dry
Digestion, languid - normalizes
Expectorant
Flu
Gas -especially with caraway
Griping - helps diminish
Milk, nursing - promotes
Mucus - clears from passages
Secretagogue

Secondary Uses:
Asthma, spasmodic - oil mixed with wine in hot water
Colic - infusion
Indigestion
Nausea
Stimulant

Other Possible Uses:
Antiseptic
Aphrodisiac
Catarrh, infantile - tea (1-3 tsp. frequently)
Childbirth - facilitates
Convulsions - safe to use
Emmenagogue
Epilepsy
Fat breakdown
Hiccups
Infection
Insomnia - a few drops with hot milk
Menopause, symptoms
Sinusitis

External Uses:
Aromatic
Bad breath
Expectorant - smoke seeds
Eyewash - soothing
Facial packs
Insects - oil with sassafras and carbolic oils

- Used to flavor liqueurs.
- Infusion: 10 - 30 grains infused in distilled water. Wineglassful doses.
- Oil: 4 - 20 drops essential oil on a sugar cube.
- Tea: ½ pint boiling water poured over 2 tsp. bruised seeds.
- Mouthwash: A few tsp. seeds boiled in 1 cup of water.
- Shock Treatment: Macerate with cloves, cinnamon, ginger and 1-1/2 cups vodka for 6 weeks. Strain and bottle.

Anise, Star

Illicium verum
Magnolia Family
Parts Used: Seeds, Oil
Habitat: China; the East; Japan.

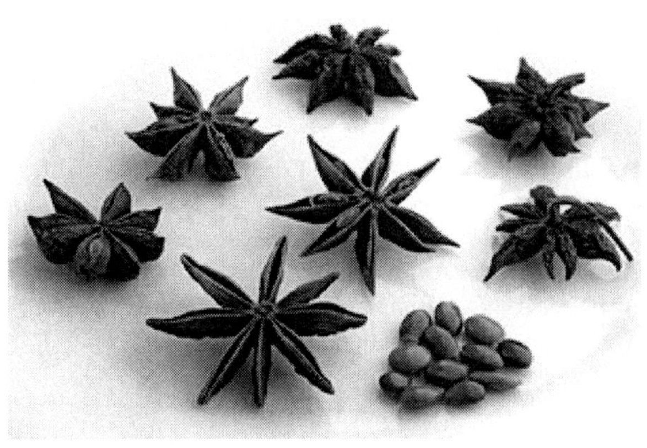

Also known as: Aniseed Stars; Badiana; Chinese Anise

Dosage: 15 - 30 grains

Primary Uses:
Spice

Secondary Uses:
Gas
Stimulant

Other Possible Uses:
Colic
Diuretic
Rheumatism

External Uses:
Aromatic

Arnica

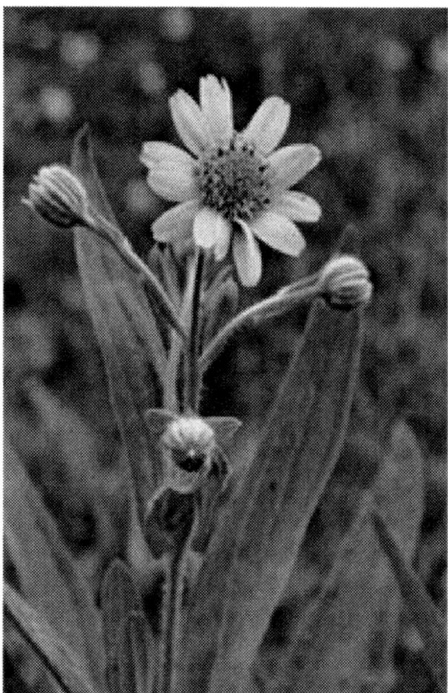

Arnica montana
Composite Family
Parts Used: Flower, Root
Habitat: Central Europe, woods and mountain pastures; England; Scotland.

Also known as: Leopard's Bane; Mountain Tobacco

Dosage: 1 - 2 grains

- Repeated external applications may cause severe inflammation.
- Never use on broken skin or open wounds.
- Irritating to the stomach - best kept external.
- **There have been numerous cases of severe poisoning and many people are especially sensitive to it. May be fatal.**
- Large doses are poisonous.
- Only use for two weeks at a time. If rash develops, discontinue use.
- **Do not use in any form during pregnancy - it contains a compound that induces labor.**

Primary Uses:
Diuretic
Stimulant

Secondary Uses:
Antibiotic
Anti-inflammatory

Other Possible Uses:
Cell growth - stimulates
Coughs
Expectorant

External Uses:
Arthritis
Bath
Bruises - reduce
Carpal Tunnel Syndrome
Feet, tender - hot footbath
Fractures
Hair, growth - applied to scalp
Inflammation, joint
Irritation, nasal passage - ointment
Lips, chapped - ointment
Muscle soreness - stops
Pain - one of the best
Skin irritation
Sprains
Swelling - reduces
Rheumatic pain
Wounds - heals

- Ointment: Heat 1 ounce of arnica with 1 ounce olive oil in water over a low flame for several hours. Strain through several layers of cheesecloth.

Arrowroot

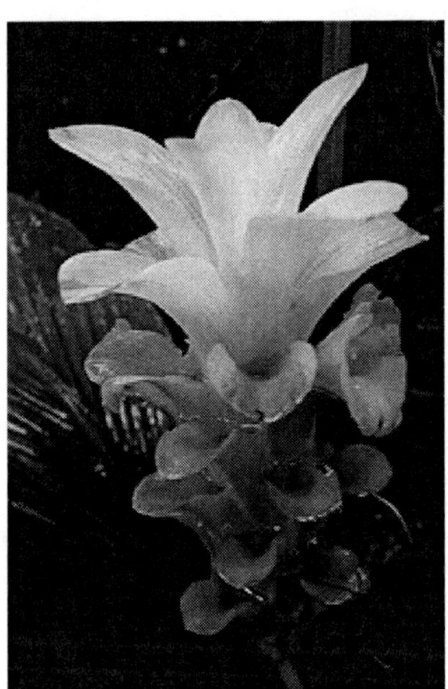

Maranta arundinaceae
Prayer Plant (Marantaceae) Family
Part Used: Starch of the rhizome
Habitat: Bengal; Central America; Java; Mauritius; Natal; Philippines; west Africa; West Indian Islands.

Also known as: Araruta; Bermuta Arrowroot; East or West Indian Arrowroot; Indian Arrowroot; Maranta Indica; Maranta ramosissima; Maranta Starch

Dosage: 20 - 60 grains

Primary Uses:
Bowel inflammation
Inflammation, internal
Infant weaning - jelled
Nutritive, especially children & invalids (easy and pleasant)

Other Possible Uses:
Plant poisons - fresh juice with water

External Uses:
Bites and stings
Gangrene

- Nourishing and easily digested for convalescents.
- Jelled Arrowroot: Make into smooth paste with a bit of cold milk or water, then slowly stir in boiling milk. May add wine, honey, etc. for flavor.

Astragalus

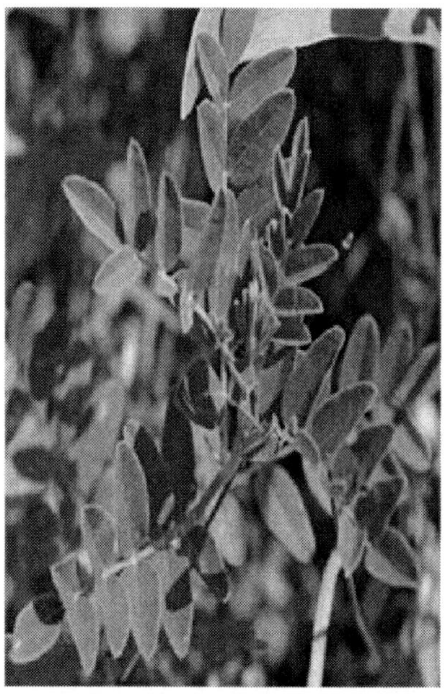

Astragalus membranaceous
Legume Family
Part Used: Root
Habitat: China; Manchuria; Mongolia; grassy hills and thickets.

Also known as: Huang-Qi; Locoweed; Mill Vetch Root; Yellow Vetch

Dosage: No recommended dosage.

- Do not use in the presence of a fever.
- Do not use in the presence of acute infection.
- Do not use with medications like Warfarin, etc. Similar compounds may cause bleeding.
- May reduce effectiveness of beta-blockers.

Primary Uses:
Cancer - prevents spread, increases white blood
cell count
Colds
Digestion - strengthens
Diuretic
Fatigue
Flu
Immune deficiency
Immune system - increases
Immune system depression from cancer treatments
Lungs, weak
Metabolism - increases
Perspiration - produces
Stamina - increases
Swollen ankles (edema)
Tumors

Secondary Uses:
AIDS
Angina, pain
Bladder infection
Burns
Diabetes & side effects, esp. with eyes
Heart - normalizes function
Heart attack - increases circulation after
Heart disease, all
Heart tissue - protects, especially after heart attack
High blood pressure
HIV
Infection, frequent
Infertility, male - helps motility
Kidneys - normalizes function
Rheumatoid arthritis

External Uses:
Antibacterial

- The taste should be sweet.
- Non-toxic.

Balm of Gilead

Commiphora Opobalsamum
Bursera Family
Part Used: Resinous Juice
Habitat: Countries around the Red Sea.

Also known as: Balessan; Balsam of Gilead; Balsam Poplar; Balsam Tree; Baune de la Mecque; Bechan; Cottonwood; Dossemo; Judiacum; Mecca Balsam; Tacamahack

Dosage: 5 - 10 grains per day

Primary Uses:
Chest complaints - tincture
Expectorant
Stimulant

Secondary Uses:
Diuretic
Kidney complaints - tincture
Urinary tract diseases

Other Possible Uses:
Antibiotic
Fever
Rheumatism
Scurvy
Stomach complaints - tincture
Tonic

External Uses:
Antiseptic
Bruises - with lard or oil
Burns - simmered with oil
Colds - shortens, ointment
Flu - shortens - ointment
Nasal salve - simmered with oil
Rheumatism, pain - simmered with oil
Sunburn - simmered with oil
Swelling - with lard or oil
Ulcers, skin, chronic
Wounds, infected

Barberry

Berberis vulgaris
Barberry Family
Parts Used: Bark, Berries, Stem, Root
Habitat: Asia, temperate; England; Europe; Ireland; northern Africa; Scotland.

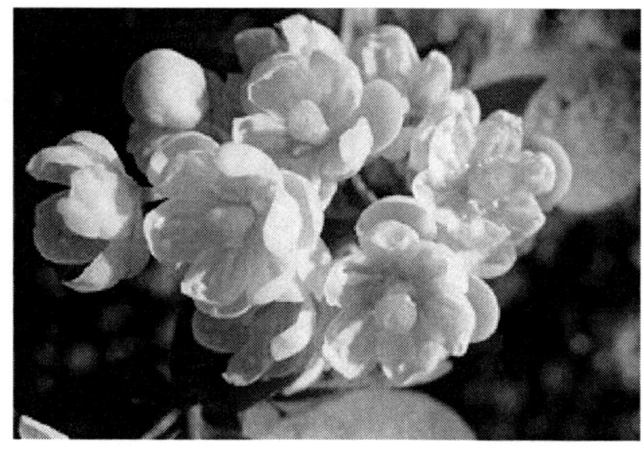

Also known as: Berberis Dumetorum; Berbery; Pipperidge Bush

Dosage: 5 - 10 grains several times a day or ¼ tsp. several times a day

- **Do not use during pregnancy or while nursing - stimulates uterine muscles.**
- Use caution with gallstones - promotes bile production.
- Do not use for food poisoning - while it does kill many microorganisms that cause food poisoning, it also slows down the motion of the intestinal tract and traps the poison and organisms inside the body.
- Men seeking to be fathers should avoid this herb - it interferes with the maturation of sperm cells.
- May lower blood sugar.
- Has tannins - may cause diarrhea and heartburn.
- Strong extracts may cause stomach upset.

Primary Uses:
Antiseptic
Biliousness
Constipation
Jaundice, all cases
Liver, derangement
Purgative - mild, larger doses
Tonic, blood

Secondary Uses:
Antibiotic (may be better than sulfa drugs) good
for antibiotic-resistant bacteria
Debility, general
Diarrhea
Digestion - regulates
Gallstones - root & stem bark
Malaria
Stomachic - tonic
Ulcers, peptic

Other Possible Uses:
Breathing - slows
Bronchial constriction
Fevers, intermittent
Heart rate - decreases
Kidney stones - preventative (stem & root bark)
Scurvy
Stimulant
Typhus

External Uses:
Abrasions - compress
Antiseptic
Astringent
Bacteria on skin - kills
Burns - reduces infection risk, compress
Cuts - compress
Cutaneous eruptions - lotion
Sore mouth - gargle
Sore throat - jelly of berries or syrup
Yeast infections (Mastitis, Candida Albicans)
Kills salmonella, staphylococcus, streptococcus, various fungi, shigella and vibrio.

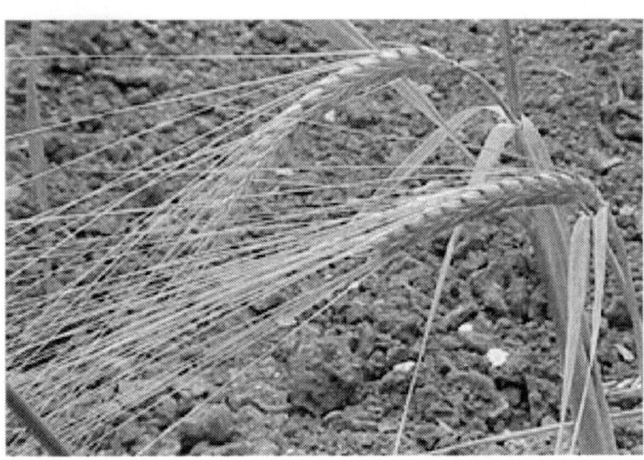

Barley Grass

Hordeum distichon
Grass Family
Part Used: Decorticated seeds
Habitat: Britain.

Also known as: Barley

Dosage: 10 parts to 100 parts water, boiled 20 minutes and strained. 1 - 4 ounce doses.

Primary Uses:
Colon disorders
Duodenal disorders
Nutritive
Stomach - heals

Other Possible Uses:
Inflammation
Pancratitis

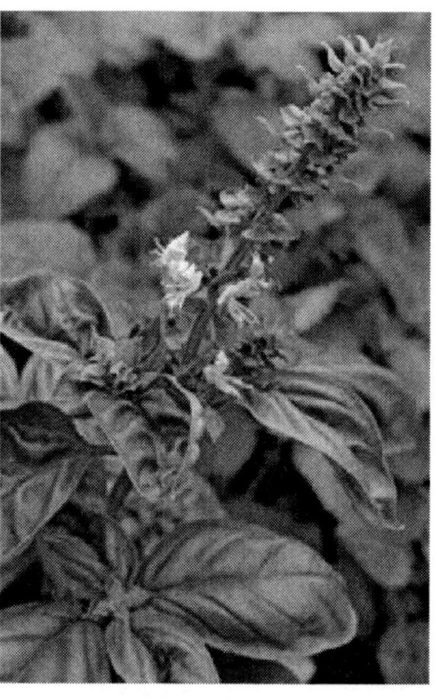

Basil

Ocymum basilium
Mint Family
Part Used: Leaves
Habitat: Worldwide.

Also known as: Albahaca; American Dittany; Saint Joseph's Wort; Sweet Basil; Witches Herb

Dosage: 30 - 60 grains

Primary Uses:
Constipation
Gas
Nausea - infusion
Rheumatism
Stomach cramps
Vomiting - infusion

Secondary Uses:
Digestion
Mother's milk
Nerves

External Uses:
Eyes, bloodshot
Flies - repels
Hives, itching
Mosquitoes - repels
Warts - seeds

- Goes well in a green salad with fresh tomatoes.

Bayberry

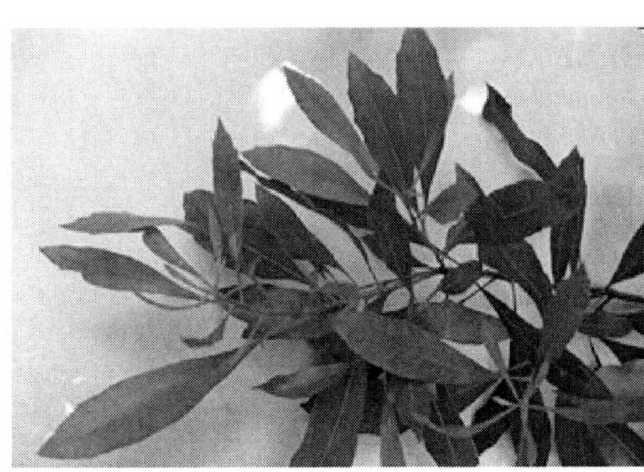

Myrica cerifera
Sweet Gale (Myricaceae) Family
Parts Used: Dried root bark, Wax
Habitat: Eastern North America in thickets near swamps and marshes and sand belt near the Atlantic coast and shores of Lake Erie.

Also known as: Candle Berry; Myrica; Tallow Shrub; Wachsgagel; Wax Myrtle

Dosage: 20 - 30 grains

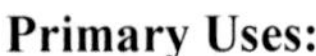

Primary Uses:
Astringent
Circulation - helps
Fever - reduces
Perspiration - produces, hot tea
Stimulant

Secondary Uses:
Colds - hot tea
Congestion - hot tea
Coughs - hot tea
Emetic - large doses (may be poisonous)
Expectorant - hot tea
Flu - hot tea
Mucus membranes, all conditions

Other Possible Uses:
Diarrhea
Hemorrhages, all kinds
Hypothyroidism
Immune system - hot tea
Jaundice
Scrofula
Tonic
Ulcers

External Uses:
Eyes
Gums, sore - wash, excellent
Hemorrhoids
Leucorrhoea
Sealing wax
Shaving lather - softening
Stimulant, indolent ulcers - poultice with elm
Throat inflammation, chronic - gargle
Uterine hemorrhage
Varicose veins, discomfort and swelling - rubbed on skin

Belladonna

Atropa Belladonna
Nightshade Family
Parts Used: Roots, Leaves, Tops
Habitat: Central and southern Europe; England; France; North America; southwest Asia; quarries and ruins.

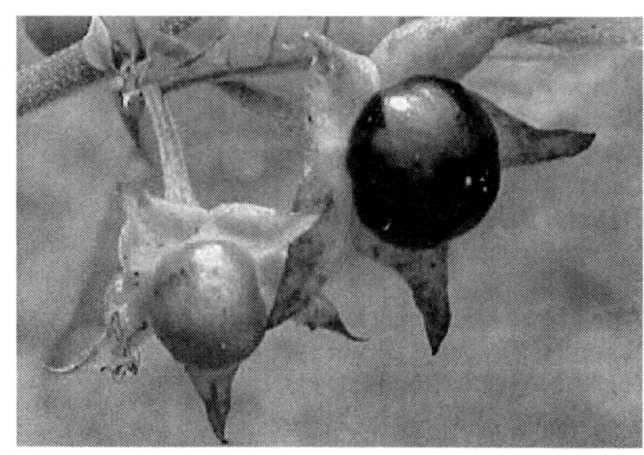

Also known as: Banewort; Black Cherry; Deadly Nightshade; Death's Herb; Devil's Cherries; Divale; Dwale; Dwaleberry; Fair Lady; Great Morel; Naughty Man's Cherries; Sorcerer's Berry; Witch's Berry

Dosage: 1/200th grain

- **POISON – do not even handle in presence of cuts or abrasions on hands or arms. (Also poisonous to cats and dogs.) Causes rapid heartbeat, hypotension, hyperthermia, confusion, hallucinations, dry mucous membranes and skin, dilated pupils that do not respond to changes in light, urine retention, seizures, coma. Death is rare.**

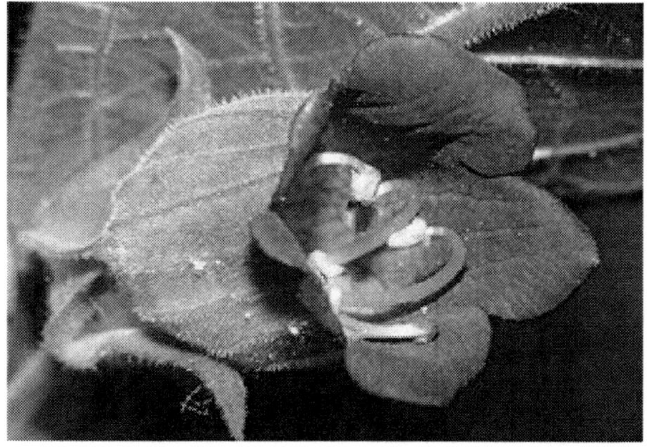

Primary Uses:
Antidote - opium, chloroform, calabur bean
Antispasmodic, asthma & colic
Diuretic
Heart - increases rate by 20-40%
Narcotic
Pneumonia
Scarlet Fever
Sedative
Sore throat, acute
Typhoid Fever

External Uses:
Backache - poultice
Dilates pupils - eye drops
Gout - poultice
Pain
Skin irritation
Antidotes:
Charcoal
Stomach pumping
Vomiting

This herb is extremely poisonous and is not recommended for use under any circumstances. It is available in pre-measured homeopathic medications, which work very well. Also, if someone is poisoned with opium, chloroform or calabur bean, take him or her to the hospital immediately. Do not try to treat them without proper medical supervision.

Bilberry (Blueberry)

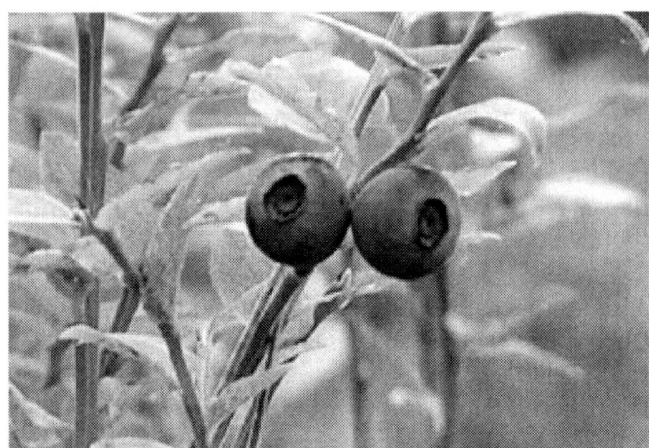

Vaccinium myrtillus
Blueberry Family
Parts Used: Fruit, Leaves (sometimes Bark)
Habitat: Barbary; Britain; Europe; Siberia; mountainous areas.

Also known as: Airelle; Black Whortles; Bleaberry; Blueberry; Huckleberry; Hurtleberry; Hurts; Trackleberry; Whinberry; Whortleberry

Dosage: 60 - 120 grains of fruit or 30 - 60 grains of leaves or bark

- Interferes with iron absorption.
- Leaves may become poisonous if taken over a long period of time.
- **Do not use during pregnancy**.
- Do not take with anticoagulants or in presence of a bleeding disorder.
- Discontinue if blood appears in urine.

Fruits:

Primary Uses:
Antiseptic, urinary tract
Astringent
Cataracts
Diarrhea - syrup (non-constipating) especially with slippery elm
Diuretic - bruised with roots & steeped in gin
Dropsy - bruised with roots & steeped in gin
Eyestrain
Gravel - bruised with roots & steeped in gin
Near-sightedness (myopia)
Night blindness
Urinary complaints
Vision, poor

Secondary Uses:
Connective tissue - strengthen & prevent degeneration
Discharges
Dysentery - syrup
Inflammation
Milk - stops
Scurvy

Other Possible Uses:
Anemia
Anxiety
Fever
Inflammation, bowel
Liver conditions
Stomach conditions
Stress

Leaves or Bark:

Primary Uses:
Diabetes - tea (leaves), must be taken for a prolonged period - reduces blood sugar directly
Eyes, general - strengthens capillaries
Insulin - controls levels

Secondary Uses:
Gout
High blood pressure
Hypoglycemia
Inflammation
Prostatitis
Rheumatoid arthritis
Ulcers, peptic

External Uses:
Mouth ulceration
Throat ulceration
Ulcers

- Prevents capillary damage in the eyes such as diabetic retinopathy, glaucoma and cataracts.
- Prevents E. coli bacteria from adhering to the linings of the bladder and intestines.

Black Cohosh

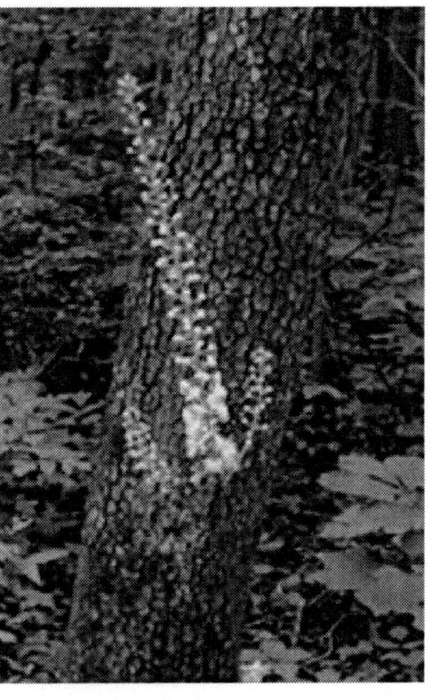

Cimicifuga racemosa
Peony Family
Part Used: Root
Habitat: North America, shady woods.

Also known as: Black Snake Root; Bugbane; Cimifuga; Squawroot

Dosage: 15 grains

- **Do not use during pregnancy (until labor) – abortive.**
- **Do not use while nursing.**
- Do not use for girls who have not reached puberty.
- Do not use with estrogen sensitive cancers (uterine, breast, etc.)
- May interfere with hormonal medications and oral contraceptives.
- Do not take with tranquilizers.
- May interfere with blood pressure medication.
- Oral antibiotics may reduce effectiveness.
- Do not overdose - large doses produce vomiting, reduced pulse, tremors and vertigo.
- May cause stomach upset - take with meals to avoid.

Primary Uses:
Asthma
Blood cleanser
Bronchitis, chronic
Coughs - stops
Diarrhea, children - small doses
Diuretic
Emmenagogue
Expectorant
High blood pressure
High cholesterol
Hot flashes
Labor - induces
Menopause, all symptoms (use minimum 8 weeks)
Morning sickness
Premenstrual Syndrome, all symptoms including migraine
Rattlesnake poisoning
Rheumatism - infusion
Sinusitis
Uterus - contracts
Whooping cough

Secondary Uses:
Arthritis
Headache
Infertility, male (motility & viability)
Leucorrhoea
Muscle spasms
Nervous system - quietens
Pain - soothes
Sedative
Tension
Vision, blurred

Other Uses:
Fever
Hysteria
Narcotic

External Uses:
Rattlesnake poison - tincture
Rheumatism

- Keep in mind that black cohosh induces labor. Using it for morning sickness has to be done in very small doses and be extremely careful.
- **Rattlesnake poisoning is nothing to risk trying to heal yourself. Herbs are no**

substitute to modern medicine for applications such as this.

- Balances hormonal levels in both men and women.
- Increases blood flow to the uterus.

Black Pepper

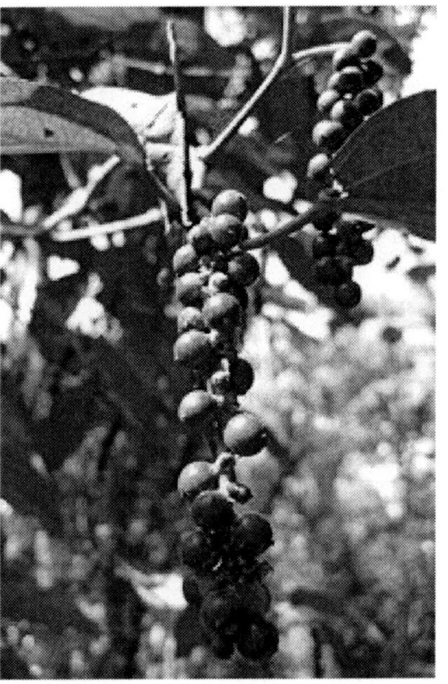

Piper nigrum
Pepper Family
Part Used: Fruit
Habitat: China; East and West Indies; Malay; Malabar; Siam; south India (wild).

Dosage: 5 - 20 grains

- Do not combine with astragalus - makes both herbs inert.

Primary Uses:
Digestion - aids, especially with meals
Gas
Spice
Stimulant, especially mucus membrane of the rectum

Secondary Uses:
Chills
Constipation - really good
Fever
Flu
Nausea
Urinary organs - stimulant
Possible Other Uses:
Arthritis
Cholera
Diarrhea
Paralysis disorders
Vertigo

External Uses:
Aromatic
Circulation - increases
Prolapsed rectum
Tongue paralysis - gargle

Black Walnut

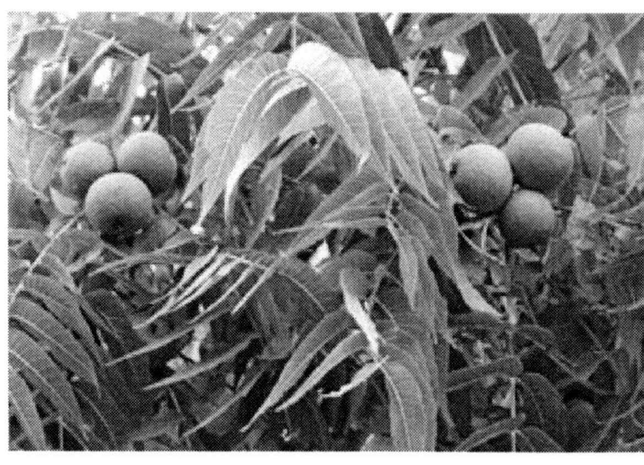

Juglans nigra
Walnut Family
Parts Used: Leaves, Bark
Habitat: Asia Minor; Britain (common walnut); Greece; Hindu-Kush to the Himalayas; India; Italy; Kashmir; Kurdon; Lebanon; Nepal; North America; Persia; Sirmore.

Also known as: Jupiter's Nuts; White Walnut

Dosage: 30 - 60 grains

Primary Uses:
Astringent - bark
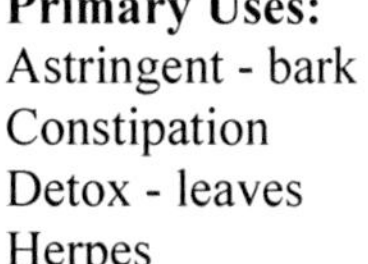
Constipation
Detox - leaves
Herpes
Laxative - very mild and effective
Perspiration - reduces
Purgative
Worms - expels

Secondary Uses:
Eczema

External Uses:
Acne
Anti-fungal
Athlete's foot
Boils
Eczema
Herpes
Mouth sores - gargle
Parasitic infection
Poison ivy
Psoriasis
Ringworm
Skin problems
Snakebite - with honey, onion and salt (to draw venom)
Sore throat - gargle
Ulcers
Warts
Worms, on lawns - destroys without harming
plants
Wounds

- The hulls have been used as a hair-coloring agent for dark hair.
- Watch out for products containing the hulls - they are a very harsh laxative. Use only the leaf.

Bladderwrack

Fucus vesiculosis
Fucaceae Family
Parts Used: Root, Stem, Leaves
Habitat: North Atlantic Ocean.

Also known as: Bladder Fucus; Black Tang; Blasentang; Cutweed; Kelp; Sea Spirit; Sea Wrack; Seetang

Dosage: 10 - 30 grains

Primary Uses:
Blood Cleanser
Obesity
Thyroid - stimulates

Secondary Uses:
Absorbs water in intestines
Kidney function
Parasites - eliminates
Worms

External Uses:
Arthritis - bruised leaves

- Take before meals for obesity.
- High in iodine.

Blessed Thistle

Carbenia benedicta
Benedictus Family
Part Used: Herb
Habitat: England; North America; southern Europe as a weed.

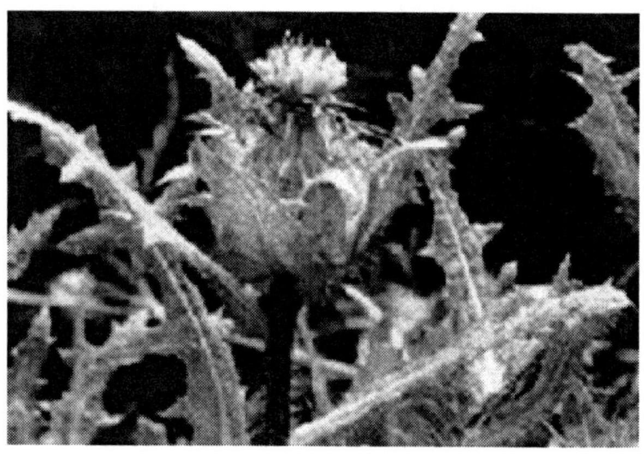

Also known as: Cricus Benedictus; Holy Thistle

Dosage: 30 - 60 grains

- **Do not use during pregnancy**.
- Emetic (very strong).

Primary Uses:
Appetite stimulant
Brain function
Circulation
Emetic - strong with little pain or inconvenience
Emmenagogue
Fever - warn infusion
Heart - strengthens
Liver
Memory
Milk - produces
Perspiration - produces
Stimulant
Tonic - cold infusion

Secondary Uses:
Bleeding - stops
Detox
Inflammation
Lungs
Stomach
Worms - leaves, dried & powdered

Other Possible Uses:
Jaundice
Kidney
Vertigo

External Uses:
Bites
Boils
Itching
Sores, festering

- Infusion: 1 ounce to 1 pint boiling water in wineglassful doses.

Blue Cohosh

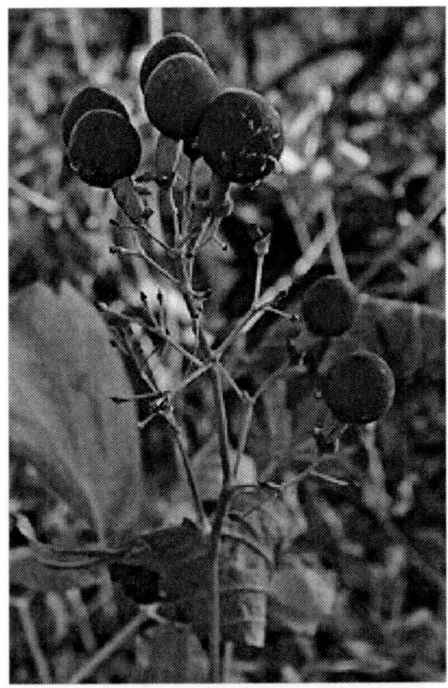

Caulophyllum thalictroides
Barberry Family
Part Used: Root
Habitat: North America, swamps and streams.

Also known as: Blueberry Root; Papoose Root; Squawroot

Dosage: 10 - 30 grains

- **Abortive.**

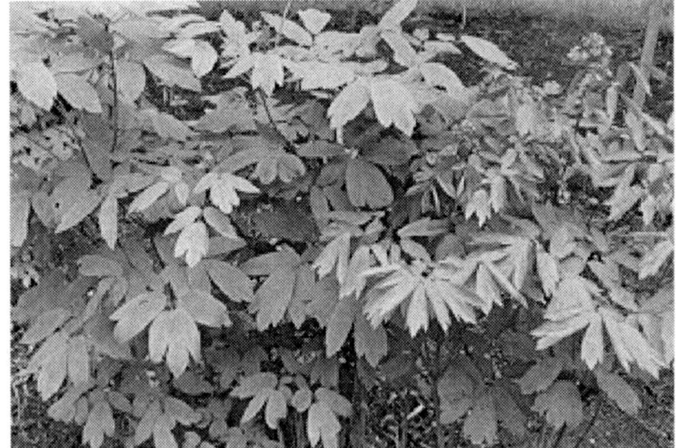

Primary Uses:
Antispasmodic, muscular
Colic
Cramps, menstrual (all disorders too)
Diabetes
Diuretic
Emmenagogue
Epilepsy
Labor - induces
Leucorrhoea
Low blood pressure
Nervous disorders
Rheumatism
Vaginitis

Secondary Uses:
Arthritis
Hysteria
Inflammation, uterine
Memory problems
Stomach cramps

Blue Vervain

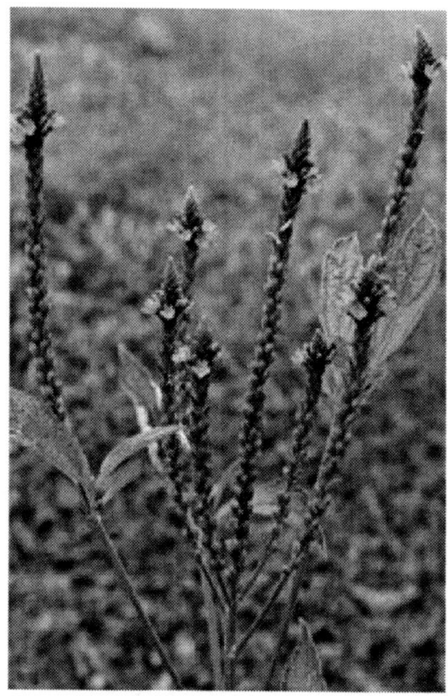

Verbena officinal; Verbena hastata
Vervain Family
Parts Used: Leaves, Flowering heads
Habitat: Barbary; China; Europe; Japan; sunny pastures and roadsides.

Also known as: Britannica; Enchanter's Plant; Herb of Enchantment; Herb of Grace; Herb of the Cross; Herba Sacra; Herba Veneris; Holy Herb; Juno's Tears; Pigeon's Grass; Pigeonweed; Simpler's Joy; Van-Van; Verbena; Vervain; Vervan

Dosage: 15 - 30 grains

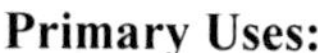

Primary Uses:
Asthma
Bladder - relieves
Colds
Coughs
Delirium
Epilepsy
Fever - reduces
Flu
Headache
Female disorders, all
Nervous complaints - preventative
Perspiration - promotes
Pneumonia
Worms

Secondary Uses:
Antispasmodic
Convulsions
Emmenagogue
Depression
Mother's milk - increases
Purgative - painless

Other Possible Uses:
Gallbladder
Genitals
Gout
Liver
Migraine
Tranquilizer - with mistletoe

External Uses:
Astringent
Headache - poultice
Inflammation - poultice
Poison ivy & oak - poultice
Rheumatism - poultice
Wounds - poultice

Boneset

Eupatorium perfoliatum
Composite Family
Part Used: Herb
Habitat: North America, low meadows and damp ground.

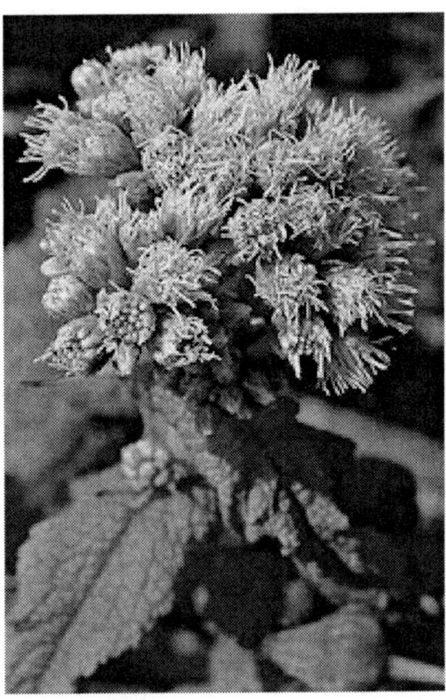

Also known as: Agueweed; Crosswort; Feverwort; Indian Sage; Sweating Plant; Teasel; Thoroughwort; Wood Boneset

Dosage: 10 - 40 grains

- Large doses are emetic and purgative.
- Do not take long term - produces toxicity.

Primary Uses:
Calms the body
Colds - preventative
Coughs
Expectorant - warm
Fever, all (one of the best)
Flu symptoms, all (one of the best)
wineglassfuls, warm every ½ hour for 4-5 hours
Laxative - cold (drink)
Perspiration - produces, warm infusion
Phlegm - loosens
Worms, intestinal

Secondary Uses:
Appetite stimulant
Detox
Emmenagogue
Indigestion - infusion
Restores normal body function

Other Possible Uses:
Anti-inflammatory
Bronchitis
Congestion
Typhoid fever
Yellow fever

Borage

Borago officinalis
Borage Family
Parts Used: Leaves and Flowers
Habitat: Europe; United States; near dwellings and rubbish heaps.

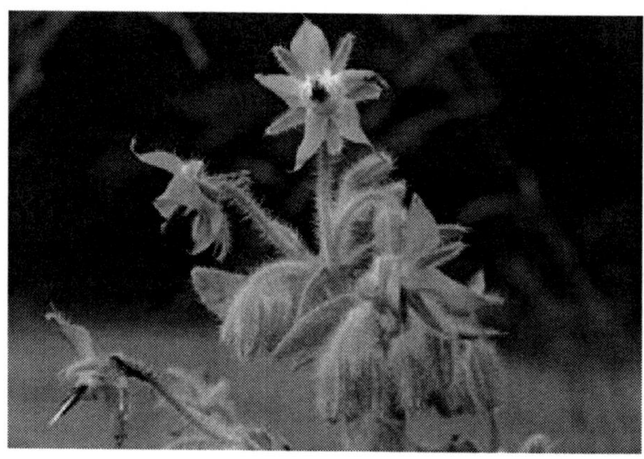

Also known as: Borrage; Bugloss; Burrage; Herb of Gladness

Dosage: 60 grains

Primary Uses:
Adrenal tonic
Jaundice
Nails - promotes healthy
Nerves, frazzled
Phlegm - clears
Premenstrual Syndrome
Sedative
Skin - promotes healthy

Secondary Uses:
Diuretic
Fever
Inflammation, internal - soothes tissue
Kidneys - promotes activity
Laxative - mild
Rheumatism

Other Possible Uses:
Chest complaints
Mother's milk - increases
Snake bite
Sore throat

External Uses:
Mouth ulcers - gargle
Swelling - poultice

- The flowers are edible, and are good for salads, floating in drinks, soups, etc.
- Plant with strawberries to help them resist disease and produce bigger fruit.
- Used in medieval times as a morale booster.
- Infusion: 1 ounce of dried leaves to 1 pint boiling water in wineglassful doses.

Buchu

Barosma betulina
Rue Family
Part Used: Leaves
Habitat: Southwest Cape Colony in South Africa.

Also known as: Bookoo; Bucoo; Buku; Diosma Betulina; Oval Buchu; Short Buchu

Dosage: 5 - 30 grains

- May irritate the kidneys.

Primary Uses:
Bladder infections & cramps
Catarrh, bladder - infusion
Cystitis
Diuretic
Gravel, bladder - infusion
Inflammation, bladder - infusion
Kidney problems - controls
Kidney stones

Secondary Uses:
Antiseptic
Digestive disorders
Inflammation, prostate
Stimulant, body

Other Possible Uses:
Colon inflammation
Diabetes
Gum inflammation
Mucous membrane inflammation
Perspiration - promotes
Vaginal inflammation

- Do not boil the leaves - it will damage them.
- Infusion: 1 ounce fresh or dried leaves to 1 pint boiling water, in wineglassful doses 3 - 4 times daily.

Burdock

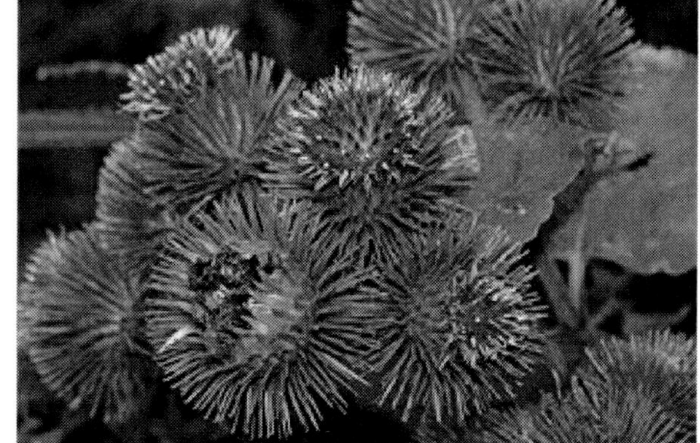

Arctium lappa
Composite Family
Parts Used: Root, Seeds, Herb
Habitat: Asia; England; Europe; North America; damp places, waste ground, old buildings, roadsides.

Also known as: Bardana; Beggar's Buttons; Burrseed; Clot-Bur; Cockle Buttons; Cockleburr; Dog Burr; Edible Burdock; Fox's Clote; Great Burdock; Greater Burdock; Happy Major; Hardock; Lappa; Hurrburr; Lappa Bardana; Love Leaves; Personata; Philanthropium; Thorny Burr; Turkey Burr

Dosage: 60 - 120 grains

- **Large quantities may stimulate uterus - use with caution during pregnancy.**

Primary Uses:
Blood cleanser - one of the best
Cancer, cell mutation (reduces)
Detox
Diabetes - seeds (valuable supplemental food)
Diuretic
Gout - tea
Kidney problems, all
Gallbladder function - restores
Immune system - stimulates
Liver function - restores
Perspiration - produces

Secondary Uses:
Arthritis
Asthma
Blood sugar - lowers, prevents surging & falling
Colds
Cystitis
Dog bites
Eczema - with yellow dock and sarsaparilla
Flu
Measles
Muscle relaxant
Rheumatism
Sciatica - tea
Scurvy
Syphilis
Tonsillitis

Other Possible Uses:
Backache

External Uses:
Balding
Boils
Bruises - poultice
Canker sores
Dandruff
Eczema
Gout - poultice
Hair loss - combats
Hemorrhoids
Insect bites
Streptococcus bacteria - kills on skin
Swelling - poultice
Tumors - poultice

- Contains chromium.
- Leaves and flowers are used in soups and salads.
- Fills intestines with fiber, blocking sugar absorption, thereby possibly regulating blood sugar and aiding in diabetes.
- Reduces swelling around joints and rids body of calcified deposits.
- Reduces absorption of toxic compounds in foods.
- There are burdock seed cereals in Japanese groceries - look for "Gobo" or "Goboshi".

Butcher's Broom

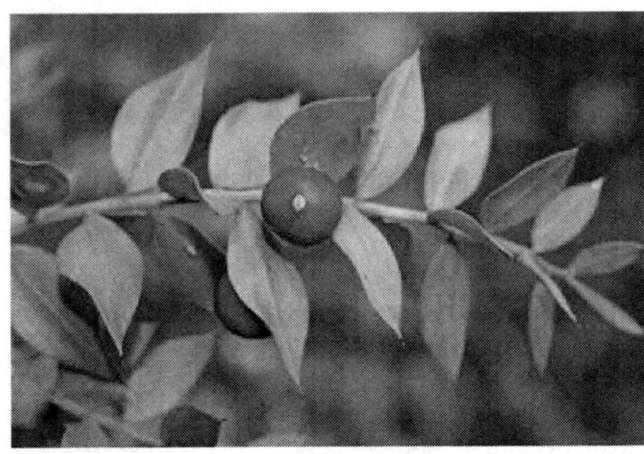

Ruscus aculeatus
Lily Family
Parts Used: Whole Plant
Habitat: South England, woods, bush and waste areas.

Also known as: Jew's Myrtle; Knee Holly; Kneeholm; Kneeholy, Pettigree; Sweet Broom

Dosage: No recommended dosage.

- Do not use in presence of high blood pressure
- Large doses may produce vomiting, purging, weakening heart, lowered nerve strength, low blood pressure, poisoning and respiratory collapse.

Primary Uses:
Bladder, inflammation - tonic
Circulation disorders, especially legs
Diuretic
Dropsy
Gravel - infusion
Hemorrhoids, burning & itching - tightens blood vessels
Inflammation, all
Jaundice - infusion
Kidneys, inflammation - tonic
Obstructions, urinary - removes
Varicose veins - reduces pain and swelling
Phlegm, chest - decoction with honey
Restless Leg Syndrome
Syphilis - reduces swollen lymph glands
Tumors, scrofulous

Secondary Uses:
Bleeding - reduces by constricting vessels
Breathing, difficult - decoction with honey
Carpal Tunnel Syndrome
Constipation

Other Possible Uses:
Arthritis, swelling and pain
Bones, broken
Menieres disease
Obesity
Perspiration - produces
Rheumatism
Vertigo

External Uses:
Hemorrhoids, pain, burning, itching
Varicose veins - cream, reduces pain & swelling during pregnancy

- Young stalks are eaten like asparagus.
- Used as brooms to sweep butchers' blocks.
- Reduces orthostatic hypotension (a drop in blood pressure when rising from sitting that causes fainting and dizziness).
- Effectiveness is increased when combined with Vitamin C.

Caraway

Carum Carvi
Carrot Family
Part Used: Seeds (Fruit)
Habitat: Asia; northern and central Europe.

Also known as: Al caravea; Carrywa; Carryways

Dosage: 30 - 60 grains

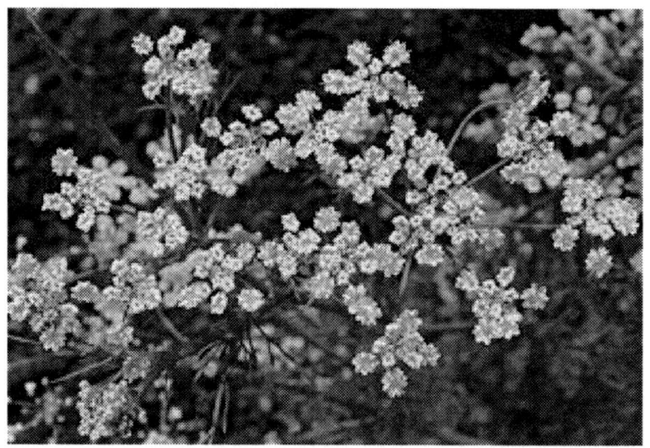

- **Do not give to infants or children except for the extract.**

Primary Uses:
Anorexia
Appetite stimulant - powerful
Gas - 1-4 drops essential oil on sugar cube or in 1 tsp. water (one of the best)

Secondary Uses:
Colic
Digestive disorders
Nausea
Stimulant
Stomachic

Other Possible Uses:
Colds - tea
Coughs - tea
Hysteria
Mother's milk - stimulates

External Uses:
Aromatic
Bruises - poultice
Toothache - oil soaked on cotton

Cascara Sagrada

Rhamnus purshiana
Buckthorn Family
Part Used: Bark
Habitat: United States, Idaho to the Pacific Ocean.

Also known as: Buckthorn; Californian Buckthorn; Sacred Bark

Dosage: 15 - 30 grains

- Do not overdose - may irritate intestines.
- Must be aged a minimum of two years or will cause severe griping and vomiting.

Primary Uses:
Bowels - tones
Gallstones
Laxative
Liver disorders

Secondary Uses:
Colitis
Leukemia
Parasites

- Cascara Sagrada is suitable for elderly persons and infants as it is very mild. It is non-habit forming and doses do not need to be increased for effectiveness.
- Works well for constipation in dogs.

Catnip

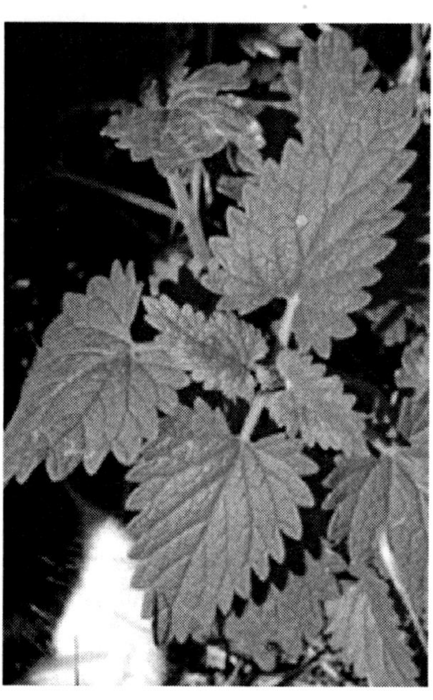

Nepeta cataria
Mint Family
Parts Used: Leaves, Herb
Habitat: Asia (temperate); central and southern England, as a weed; Europe; Ireland; North America; Scotland.

Also known as: Catmint; Catnep; Cat's Play; Cat's Toy

Dosage: 30 - 60 grains

- Always infuse - boiling spoils it.
- Very volatile - cover up, especially when infusing.
- Large doses of the warm tea act as an emetic.

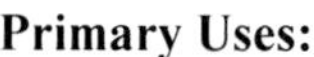

Primary Uses:
Antispasmodic
Appetite stimulant
Colds
Colic
Convulsions
Digestion, disturbances - tea
Diuretic
Emmenagogue - cold juice of plant
Fever - reduces
Flu - tea
Gas - expels
Infectious childhood diseases
Inflammation
Insanity
Insomnia, without affecting the body the next day
Nerves
Nightmares
Pain
Perspiration - promotes without increasing body heat
Restlessness
Sedative - mild (induces relaxation)
Tonic

Secondary Uses:
Antimicrobial
Bronchitis
Chicken Pox - reduces eruptions
Cramps, menstrual
Diarrhea
Measles - reduces eruptions
Miscarriage - preventative
Morning sickness
Premature birth - preventative
Upset stomach

External Uses:
Fever - tea enema, reduces quickly
Hair growth - encourages
Inflammation - poultice

- Enemas are safe for children for reducing fever.
- Relaxes tight muscles.
- Moves food and infections out of the digestive tract.
- Attracts bees and cats.
- Rubbed on raw meat as a tenderizer.

Cat's Claw

Uncaria tomentosa
Madder Family (same as coffee)
Part Used: Bark
Habitat: South and Central America, especially Amazon rain forest.

Also known as: Una De Gato

Dosage: No guidelines

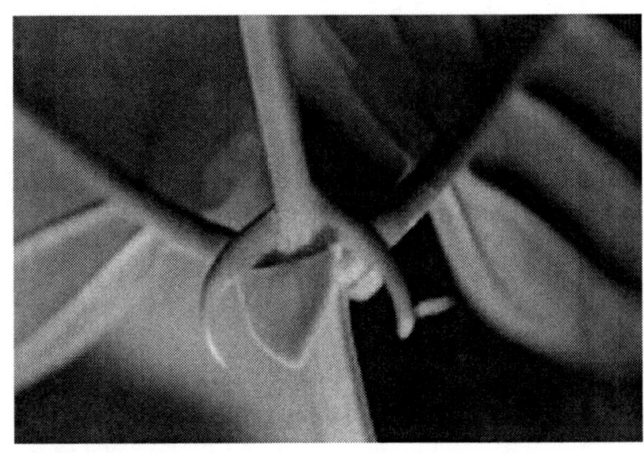

- **Do not take during pregnancy - abortive.**
- **Do not use while nursing.**
- Do not use with insulin.
- Do not use in presence of a bone marrow transplant - may cause rejection of the transplant.
- Do not use in presence of organ transplants - may cause rejection.
- Do not use in presence of a graft versus host disease.
- May cause possible rejection of foreign tissue.

Primary Uses:
Anti-inflammatory
Antioxidant - especially during chemotherapy
& radiation treatments
Arthritis, all forms
Cancer
Immune system - enhances
Tumors
Ulcers
Viral infections

Secondary Uses:
AIDS
Asthma
Colds
Detox, intestinal tract - replenishes friendly bacteria
Diabetes
Gastritis
Herpes
HIV
Lyme Disease
Rheumatism
Urinary tract inflammation

- Used in South America as a contraceptive.
- Balances the correct number of macrophages. Increases white blood cell count if below 4000 but decreases if above 9000.
- Helps the body to produce T-cells and white blood cells in normal numbers.
- Both saliva and the tongue negate this herb. Take in a capsule or with plenty of water when using a tincture to get it past the tongue for absorption.
- Potency is increased when used in conjunction with lemon or vinegar.
- May stop mutation of cells in long-term smokers.

Cayenne

Capsicum minimum
Nightshade Family
Part Used: Fruit (ripe and dried)
Habitat: Zanzibar; other tropical and sub-tropical countries.

Also known as: African Pepper; Bird Pepper; Capsicum; Chili; Chili Pepper; Chilies; Red Pepper

Dosage: 1 - 10 grains

- Irritating to hemorrhoids.
- Excessive use may damage liver or kidneys.
- Never use on broken skin.
- In external use, capsaicin cream should never be applied to broken skin, eyes, or mucous membranes.

Primary Uses:
Alcoholism - reduces dilated blood vessels and
relieves chronic congestion
Appetite stimulant
Colds
Digestion - promotes
Gas - relieves
Hangover
Heart
High blood pressure
Indigestion
Lungs, possibly cancer within
Metabolism
Nausea
Perspiration - stimulates
Stimulant - one of the strongest
Stomach
Ulcers

Secondary Uses:
Anti-inflammatory
Anti-irritant
Arthritis
Asthma
Diabetes
Food poisoning*
Heat stress**
Obesity - increases metabolism
Rheumatism
Sinusitis
Sore throat
Other Possible:
Migraine

External Uses:
Arthritis
Circulation - increases
Diabetic nerve damage - cream
Herpes, nerve damage - cream
Pain
Psoriasis
Sore muscles

*Sterilizes foods against the effects of the following bacterial contaminants: Bacillus subtilis, Clostridium, Sporogenes, Tetani and Streptococcus Pyogenes.

**Hot peppers give heat resistance when consumed, by dilating blood vessels, allowing cooling of the blood and stimulating perspiration.

- Cayenne is available in capsules as both regular and "cool" in which the "hot" aspect of the pepper has been removed or buffered.
- Some studies suggest that capsaicin reduces the carcinogenic effects of certain air pollutions by reducing the liver's production of enzymes necessary to activate environmental contaminants.
- This substance is almost impossible to remove from contact lenses.
- Added to herbal teas, increases absorption and action of other herbs.

Centuary

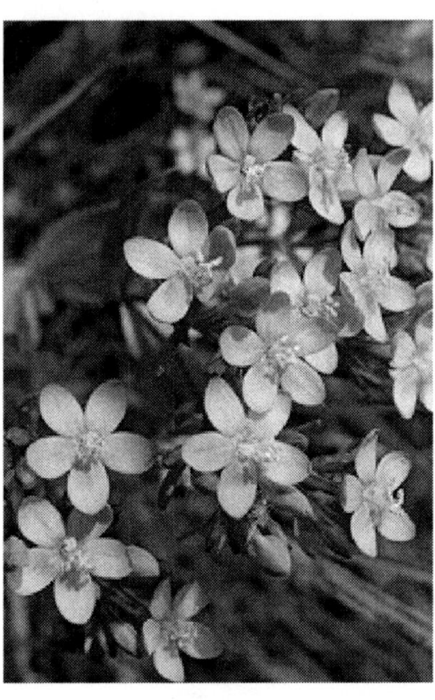

Erythraea centaurium
Gentian Family
Parts Used: Herbs and Leaves
Habitat: Europe; north Africa; dry pastures and cliffs.

Also known as: Centaury Gentian; Centory; Century; Christ's Ladder; Feverwort; Filwort; Gentian; Red Centaury

Dosage: 30 - 60 grains

- **Do not take during pregnancy.**

Primary Uses:
Appetite stimulant
Detox
Fever, intermittent
Stomachic
Tonic

Secondary Uses:
Bitter
Digestion, languid
Gout
Rheumatism, muscular
Worms

Other Possible Uses:
Colic - decoction
Dropsy
Emmenagogue
Heartburn
Indigestion
Jaundice - with barberry bark
Kidneys
Labor pain
Liver
Perspiration - produces
Throat, sore

External Uses:
Aromatic
Freckles
Sores - cleanses
Spots
Ulcers - closes
Wounds

Chamomile

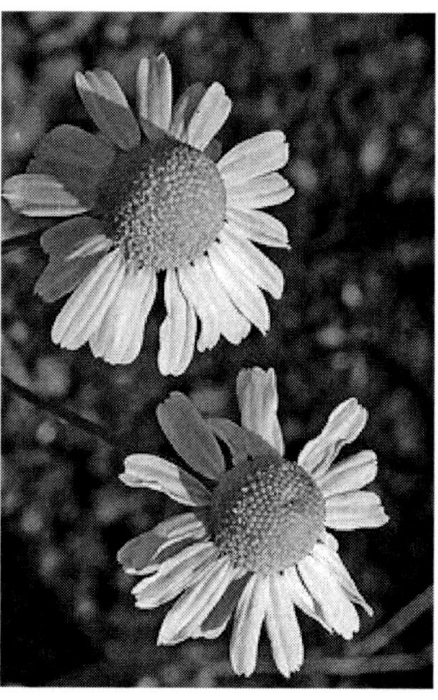

Anthemis nobilis (common); Matricaria chamomilla (German)
Composite Family
Part Used: Flowers
Habitat: Asia, temperate; Europe; Great Britain; north Africa; cornfields.

Also known as: Camomyle; Chamaimelon; German Chamomile; Ground Apple; Manzanilla; Maythen; Roman Chamomile; Whig Plant; Wild Chamomile

Dosage: 30 - 60 grains

- Do not use if allergic to ragweed.
- Contains natural blood thinners (coumarins). Avoid taking with Warfarin, which is similar.
- Increases the effect of Valium.

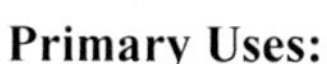

Primary Uses:
Antibacterial
Antihistamine
Anti-inflammatory
Anxiety
Appetite stimulant
Arthritis
Asthma
Bladder problems
Colds
Colitis
Cramps, menstrual
Digestion
Diuretic
Diverticulitis
Fever
Gas
Headache
Hemorrhoids
Indigestion
Infantile convulsions
Insomnia
Jaundice
Muscle cramps
Nerves & nervous disorders
Pain, back
Premenstrual Syndrome
Rheumatism
Sedative
Sleep
Stomach cramps, disorders & nervous
Stress
Tonic
Tranquilizer
Ulcers, peptic - protects & treats
Worms

Secondary Uses:
Allergies
Antioxidant
Antispasmodic
Arteriosclerosis
Attention Deficit Disorder
Colic
Irritable Bowel Syndrome
Lupus
Menstrual irregularities
Morning sickness - with ginger
Muscle spasms - preventative

Other Possible Uses:
Alcohol D.T.'s
Brain fatigue
Cancer, endometrial
Eyes
Heart
Kidneys, stones
Perspiration - produces
Spleen - with sugar
Smoking - quitting
Tissue

External Uses:
Abrasions - cream (reduces weeping of fluids)
Antibacterial

Anti-fungal - with vinegar (on skin)
Anti-inflammatory
Cuts - cream (reduces weeping of fluids)
Dental problems
Diaper rash - cream
Douche & genital wash
Ear pain
Eczema - cream
Firms tissue - bath
Hair brightener - highlights blonde & golden tones
Hemorrhoids
Hives
Inflammation, skin
Insect repellent, especially flies
Pain in joints
Perspiration odor
Sunburn
Swelling in joints
Toothache

- Oil - beat with olive oil and steep for 24 hours. Strain.
- Effects are cumulative. Give at least 3 - 4 weeks before deciding if effective.
- Keeps a garden healthy when planted in one.

Chaste Tree

Agnus castus
Verbena Family
Part Used: Berries
Habitat: Shores of the Mediterranean.

Also known as: Monk's Pepper; Vitex

Dosage: 1 - 4 mg

Primary Uses:
Estrogen replacement therapy
Hormone balancer
Menopause
Premenstrual Syndrome

Secondary Uses:
Anaphrodesiac
Pain, limbs
Paralysis - relief
Tumors, fibroid
Weakness

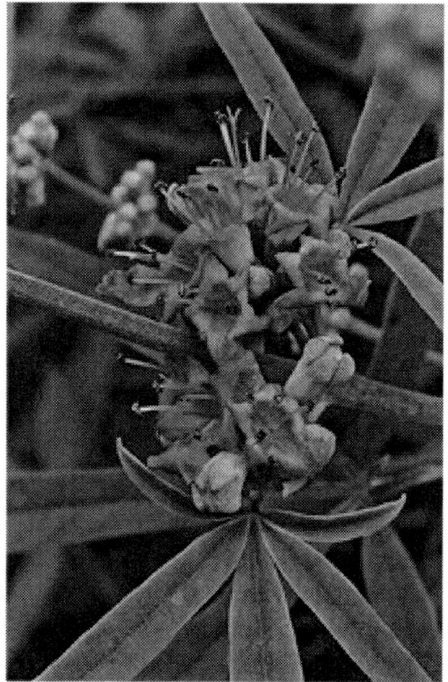

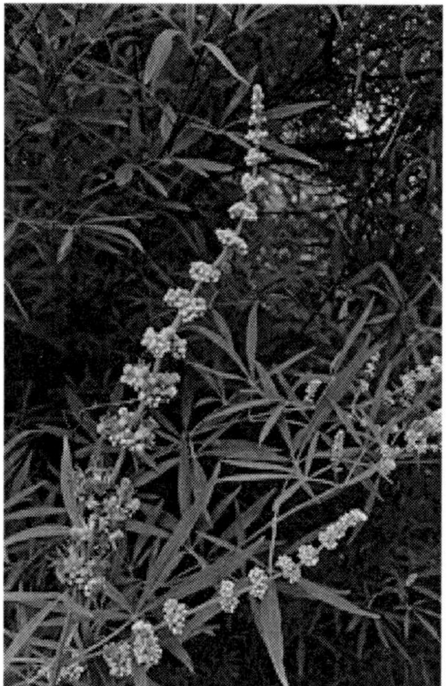

Chickweed

Stellaria media
Pink Family
Part Used: Herb
Habitat: Worldwide.

Also known as: Adder's Mouth; Indian Chickweed; Passerina; Satinflower; Star Chickweed; Starweed; Starwort; Stellaire; Stitchwort; Tongue Grass; Winterweed

Dosage: 30 - 60 grains

Primary Uses:
Bronchitis
Coughs - infusion
Hoarseness - infusion
Inflammation, internal
Lungs, mucus buildup
Obesity - old wives' remedy

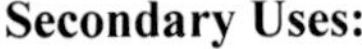

Secondary Uses:
Antacid
Bowels
Constipation - fresh decoction
Cools the body
Digestive system
Hydrophobia - with elecampane
Scurvy - juice

Other Possible Uses:
Circulatory problems
Colds
Convulsions
Cramps
Detox
Diuretic
Kidney
Palsy
Testes, swollen

External Uses:
Abscess - poultice in muslin (one of the best)
Bruises
Carbuncles - poultice in muslin (one of the best)
Eczema
Eyes, hot and red - juice
Inflammation - poultice
Irritation
Ophthalmia (moon blindness) - ointment
Piles - ointment
Sores - cools, ointment
Ulcers, indolent - poultice
Warts

- Ointment: Chop plant and boil in lard.

Cinnamon

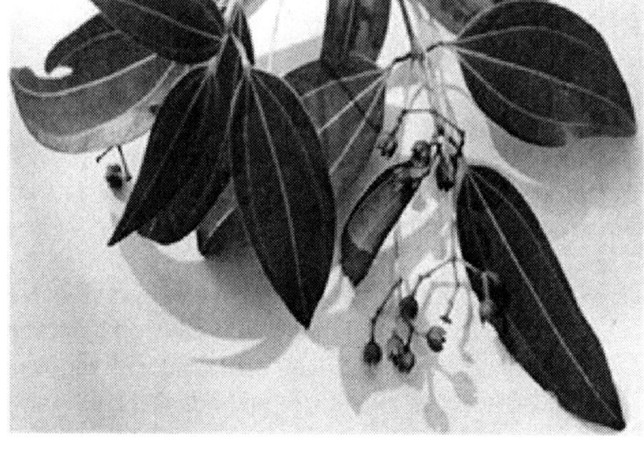

Cinnamomum zeylanicum
Laurel Family
Part Used: Bark
Habitat: Brazil; Ceylon; Cochin-China; Eastern Islands; India; Jamaica; Malabar; Mauritius; Sumatra.

Also known as: Cassia; Cinnamon Bark; Cinnamon Twig; Sweetwood

Dosage: 10 - 20 grains

- **Do not use large amounts during pregnancy.**
- The oil is toxic internally - never ingest cinnamon oil. It causes nausea, vomiting and kidney damage.
- Oil is irritating to the skin.
- May increase blood pressure.
- Avoid in presence of prostate problems.

Primary Uses:
Circulation - stimulates
Diarrhea - with chalk or charcoal
Digestion - warming
Gas
Indigestion
Nausea
Stimulant
Vomiting

Secondary Uses:
AIDS
Aphrodisiac
Cramps, menstrual
Diabetes
Fat metabolism
Fungal infection
Heart attack - prevent
HIV
Obesity
Oral thrush - tea or tincture
Stomach
Ulcers, peptic - stops without interfering with production of gastric acid
Uterine hemorrhaging - with chalk, reduces bleeding while stimulating blood flow from uterus
Yeast infection - tea or tincture
Other:
Cancer, liver - stops growth
Colds
Melanoma - stops growth

External Uses:
Antiseptic
Astringent
Embalming

- The bark is cut and allowed to ferment in the field before drying.
- Chewing on a stick of cinnamon is said to relieve a nose cold.
- Drinking cinnamon daily is said to aid cold hands and feet.

Cloves

Eugenia caryophyllata
Clove Family
Part Used: Undeveloped Flower
Habitat: Molucca Islands; southern Philippines.

Dosage: 5 - 10 grains

- Do not use the pure essential oil internally.
- Oil is an irritant - dilute with olive oil before use.
- Do not use oil for pain associated with root canal work - may cause inflammation.
- Do not give to children under 6 years old - may cause gastric upset.

Primary Uses:
Digestion
Gas - alleviates pressure, oil
Indigestion
Nausea - powdered or infusion
Parasites
Teeth - oil
Vomiting - oil (two drops in 1 cup water)

Secondary Uses:
Bronchitis
Cancer, stomach - oil (protects against)
Food poisoning - oil*
Headache

Other Possible Uses:
Aphrodisiac
Detox
Dreams
Eyes
Melancholia
Memory
Stimulant

External Uses:
Analgesic
Anti-fungal
Anti-inflammatory
Antimicrobial
Antiseptic - powerful
Germicide - strong
Insects - repels
Mouthwash
Toothache – oil

*Clove oil kills the following bacteria: Pseudomonas aeruginosa, all species of Shigella, Staphylococcus aureus and Streptococcus pneumoniae.

- Clove tea is great to drink during labor - calms the stomach and helps with the labor.
- The oil is applied to decayed teeth for pain.

- Four Thieves Vinegar:
  - This is one version of the recipe used by the thieves during the great plague of France so they could safely rob dead bodies without fear of infection. It worked until they were caught.
  - 1 tsp. each ground clove, cinnamon and nutmeg
  - 2 tsp each dried rosemary, peppermint and sage
  - 2 tsp. crushed garlic
  - 1 liter cider vinegar
  - Put all ingredients in tightly covered glass jar and set out in strong sunlight for 15 days. Strain and bottle.

Coltsfoot

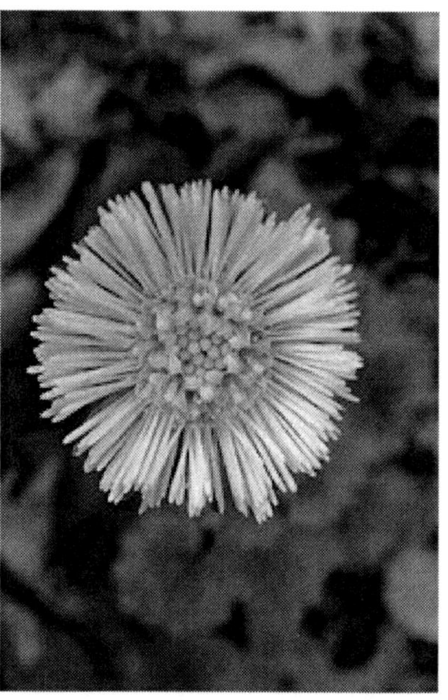

Tussilago Farfara
Composite Family
Parts Used: Leaves, Flowers, Root
Habitat: England, especially on side of railway banks and in waste areas.

Also known as: Ass's Foot; British Tobacco; Bullsfoot; Butterbur; Cough Herb; Coughwort; Donnhove; Fieldhove; Foals Foot; Foalswort; Fool's Foot; Hallfoot; Horsehoof; Tussilago

Dosage: 60 grains

- Produces liver tumors in rats.
- Do not give to children in an over-the-counter cold remedy.
- Tincture may aggravate high blood pressure.

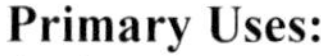

Primary Uses:
Asthma - tea or smoke with eyebright, buckbean, betony, rosemary, thyme, lavender & chamomile (British Herb Tobacco)
Bronchitis
Congestion
Coughs - smoke leaves
Coughs - juice with marshmallow root & horehound (one of the best)
Expectorant
Inflammation, internal - soothes
Lungs
Phlegm - loosens
Pneumonia
Tonic
Wheezing - juice or syrup

Secondary Uses:
Breath, shortness - juice or syrup
Colds - decoction or tea
Laryngitis

Other Possible Uses:
Diarrhea
Fever
Giddiness
Headache
Spasms
Tuberculosis
Tissues - promotes healing
Ulcers

External Uses:
Skin ailments - poultice
Skin - cooling, poultice

- Decoction: 1 ounce leaves in 1 quart water boiled down to 1 pint, sweetened with honey, in tsp. doses frequently.
- Small doses open bronchial passages while large doses close them.
- If you are concerned about liver cancer, look for "certified pyrrolizidine free" on the label, which is genetically engineered to be without the constituent that causes liver cancer. (Although, the regular herb actually only contains 1/100th of the amount that produces toxicity.) The tinctures do contain 10 times the alkaloids as the teas made with the same amount of the herb. Genetically engineered plants are harming the environment in so many ways, so please think carefully before using and promoting a genetically engineered plant of any kind. Find an alternative instead if at all possible.
- Coats the throat, relieving irritation.

Comfrey

Symphytum officionale
Borage Family
Parts Used: Roots, Leaves. All above ground parts are reliably non-toxic. Root may be toxic.
Habitat: England; Europe; temperate Asia; on banks of rivers and ditches and watery places in general.

Also known as: All-Heal; Ass Ear; Blackwort; Boneset; Bruisewort; Common Comfrey; Consolida; Consound; Gum Plant; Healing Herb; Knitback; Knitbone; Miracle Herb; Slippery Root; Wallwort; Yalluc

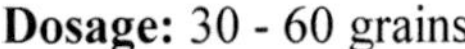

Dosage: 30 - 60 grains

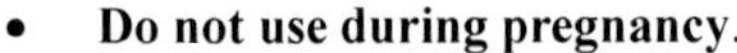

- **Do not use during pregnancy**.
- Do not use more than 3 months at a time.
- Do not take root internally - it has alkaloids that are linked to liver and lung cancer.
- Do not use with regular alcohol consumption.
- Do not use with antibiotics, Prozac, Cyclosporine, cholesterol reducing medications, calcium channel blockers for high blood pressure or any steroids.
- Do not administer to infants - either internally or externally.

Primary Uses:
Anti-inflammatory
Asthma
Astringent
Broken bones
Cell growth - stimulates
Coughs
Cramps
Diarrhea
Dysentery
Expectorant
Internal hemorrhaging, all - strong tea every two hours
Internal inflammation - soothes
Internal ulcers
Liver ulcers
Lung bleeding, coughing up blood
Lungs, all problems
Pain
Ruptures
Stomach ulcers
Tuberculosis
Whooping cough

Secondary Uses:
Blood cleanser
Catarrh
Irritable Bowel Syndrome
Rheumatoid arthritis

Other Possible Uses:
Breasts
Colds
Gout
Intestines
Phlegm - loosens

External Uses:
Abscesses
Astringent
Bedsores
Boils
Broken bones
Bruises
Burns
Cuts
Dermatitis
Douche
Gangrene in wounds – hot poultice
Hair, dry
Hemorrhoids
Insect bites - speeds healing
Pain
Psoriasis

Rash
Skin - bath
Sprains
Stings
Sunburn
Swelling
Varicose veins - compress
Warts
Wounds puss filled- speeds healing

- In severe hemorrhaging, mix tea with 1 tsp. witch hazel extract. It is very good with marshmallow root. Of course, this is not a substitute for seeing a physician for hemorrhaging as this may be life threatening.
- A traditional European May Day salad is comfrey leaves.
- Helps cells proliferation.
- Infusion is great for washing the face - promotes healthy tissue and softens the skin.

Corn Silk

Zea Mays
Haygrass Family
Part Used: Flower Pistils
Habitat: Sub-tropical and warm-climate countries worldwide.

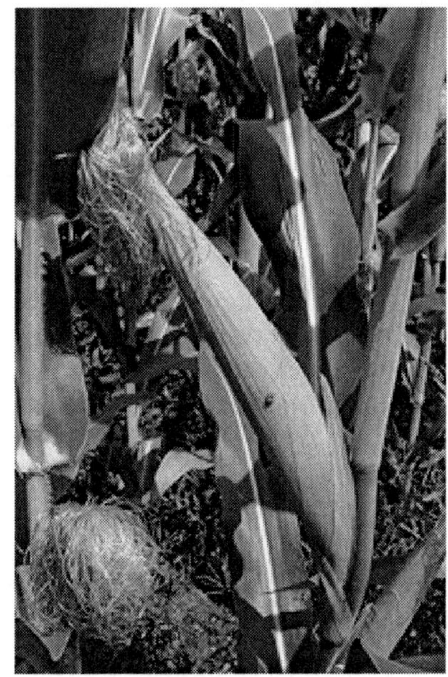

Also known as: Giver of Life; Indian Corn; Maidis Stigma; Maize; Maize Silk; Sacred Mother; Seed of Seeds; Zea

Dosage: no guidelines

- Do not take with Accupril or Quinapril - may cause excessive potassium levels, causing heart flutter, muscle twitches and atrial fibrillation.

Primary Uses:
Bedwetting - with agrimony, tea
Bladder, irritation & inflammation
Diuretic
Gravel
Inflammation, internal - soothes
Kidneys, inflammation
Stones

Secondary Uses:
Cystitis, acute & chronic
Dropsy
Gonorrhea - tea
Liver disorders
Mucus in urine - removes
Prostate disorders & enlarged
Stimulant - mild
Uric acid retention

Other Possible Uses:
Carpal Tunnel Syndrome
Detox
Hypertension
Nausea
Obesity
Premenstrual Syndrome
Small intestine - aids
Vomiting

- Rich in potassium.
- Corn water: (good for nausea and vomiting.) Bake 1 cup corn kernels at 120° until parched and dehydrated. Put in a pot and add 3-¾ cups water, reducing to 1/8 cup. Take 1 tsp. when needed or drink 1-3 tsp. in a cup of water.

Couch Grass

Agropyrum repens
Haygrass Family
Parts Used: Rhizome and Seeds
Habitat: Australia; Europe and Britain; northern Asia; North and South America; fields and waste areas.

Also known as: Dog Grass; Quackgrass; Quick Grass; Scotch Quelch; Twitch Grass

Dosage: 60 - 120 grains

Primary Uses:
Bladder disease & inflammation
Diuretic - infusion
Gravel - relieves
Kidney, disease & inflammation
Inflammation - internal, soothes
Urinary irritation & inflammation

Secondary Uses:
Bronchitis - coats inflamed surfaces
Cirrhosis - juice of roots, drunk frequently
Detox
Expectorant
Jaundice - juice of roots, drunk frequently
Laryngitis

Other Possible Uses:
Cystitis
Gout
Rheumatism

- Infusion: 1 ounce to 1 pint boiling water - taken frequently.
- Makes dogs vomit when they chew the leaves.

Cramp Bark

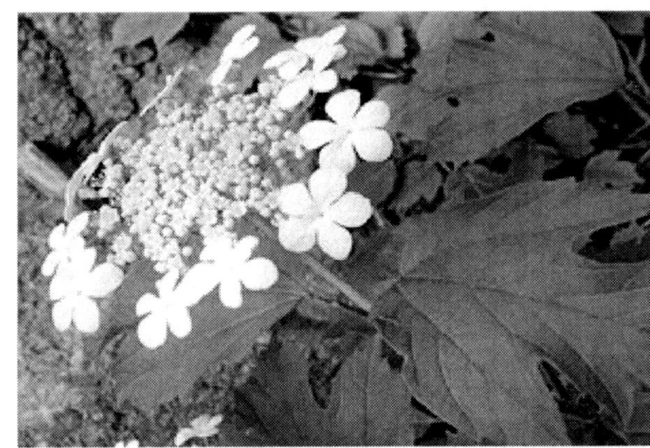

Viburnum opulus
Elder Family (some sources claim honeysuckle family)
Part Used: Bark
Habitat: England and Scotland in copses and hedgerows; eastern United States in low grounds.

Also known as: Black Haw; Dog Rowan Tree; Gaitre Berries; Guelder Rose; High Cranberry; King's Crown; May Rose; Red Elder; Silver Bells; Snowball Tree; Water Elder; Whitsun Bosses; Whitsun Rose

Dosage: 30 - 60 grains

Primary Uses:
Asthma - antispasmodic
Convulsions
Cramps, all
Fits
Heart disease
Heart palpitations
Hysteria - antispasmodic
Lockjaw
Nerves
Rheumatism
Spasms, all

Secondary Uses:
Menopause
Menstrual irregularity
Muscle relaxant

Other Possible Uses:
Anti-abortive
Miscarriage - preventative
Pregnancy pains
Tones uterus

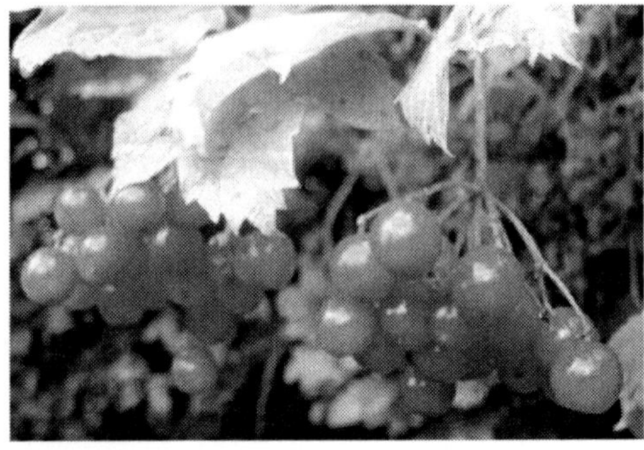

Cranberry

Vaccinium macrocarpon
Blueberry Family
Part Used: Berry
Habitat: North America, boggy regions.

Dosage: No guidelines

Primary Uses:
Bladder - prevents bacteria from attaching
Cystitis
Diuretic
Kidney infections, chronic
Urinary infections

Secondary Uses:
Internal inflammation
Muscular contractions, cramps & spasms

Other Possible Uses:
Hysteria
Nerves

- Only use pure unsweetened juice for bladder infections. The sugar in commercial juices cancels out the effectiveness and actually aggravates the infection.
- Safe to take during pregnancy and while nursing.

Damiana

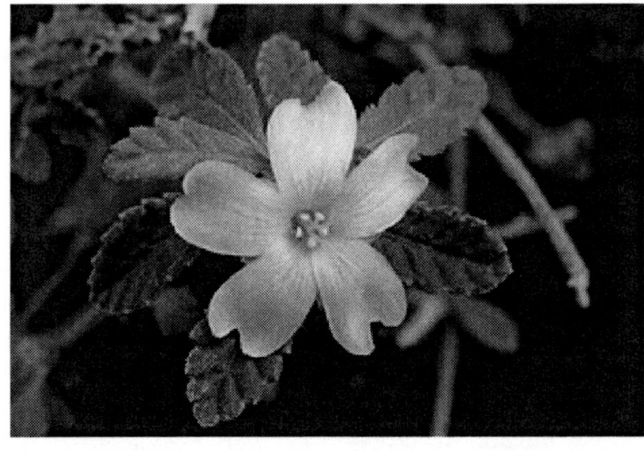

Turnera aphrodisiaca
Damiana Family
Part Used: Leaves (when plant is in flower)
Habitat: Mexico; South America; Texas; West Indies.

Also known as: Mexican Damiana

Dosage: 30 - 60 grains

- Large doses may interfere with iron absorption and many common medications. This may be avoided by adding one teaspoon of lemon to the water in which the tincture is taken.
- May lower blood sugar - use with caution in presence of diabetes.

Primary Uses:
Aphrodisiac
Bedwetting
Constipation
Depression - natural monoamine oxidase inhibitor
Digestion
Diuretic
Headache
Hypoglycemia
Impotency
Infertility, male & female - also increases sperm count
Kidneys - clears
Laxative
Lethargy
Purgative - mild
Stimulant
Tonic - general

Secondary Uses:
Anxiety
Brain tonic
Bronchitis
Emphysema
Hot flashes
Menopause
Parkinson's Disease
Urinary tract infections

- Has a cumulative effect.
- Used to treat sexual trauma, lack of desire and pleasure, and impotence. It must be used for several months for desired effect.

Dandelion

Taraxacum officinale
Composite Family
Parts Used: Leaves, Flowers, Root
Habitat: All northern hemisphere temperate zones, pastures, meadows, waste areas.

Also known as: Blow Ball; Cankerwort; Lion's Tooth; Piss-a-Bed; Priest's Crown; Puffball; Swine's Snout; White Endive; Wild Endive

Dosage: 60 - 120 grains

- Use no longer than six weeks at a time.
- May increase stomach acidity.
- Avoid during antibiotic treatment, especially with Cipro, Floxin, Maxaquin, Noroxin, and Penetrex. It may lessen their effect.
- Avoid in the presence of gallstones - increases the flow of bile. Use only as a preventative - not if already present.
- Increases potassium levels.

Primary Uses:
Abscesses
Age spots - preventative
Anemia
Appetite stimulant
Blood cleanser
Boils
Breast tumors
Cirrhosis
Constipation
Cramps
Digestion
Diuretic
Gallbladder disease
Gallstones - preventative
Glandular tonic
Gout
Hepatitis
Jaundice
Kidney disorders
Laxative - without diarrhea
Liver - cleans
Liver, sluggish from alcohol & poor diet, congestion
Rheumatism
Scurvy
Spleen
Stimulant
Stomach
Tumors

Secondary Uses:
Detox
Eczema
High blood pressure
High cholesterol
Hypochondria
Irritable Bowel Syndrome - take for 15 days minimum
Obesity - metabolizes fat, prevents hypoglycemia, regulates blood sugars, increases bile flow (Use 1 month minimum.)
Osteoporosis
Premenstrual Syndrome

Other Possible Uses:
Bowels
Eyes
Fever - reduces
Insomnia
Rids body of salt
Sleep

External Uses:
Boils
Corns
Eczema
Skin, itchy - bath
Warts - sap
Wounds

- The roasted root may be used as a coffee substitute.
- Pick leaves for a tonic salad in early spring.
- For medicinal purposes, pick leaves in early summer before the flowers bloom.
- For the best concentration in the root, wait until the plant is two years old and dig it up in the fall.
- Gall stone recipe: In 2 quarts water place one ounce each dandelion root, parsley root, balm herb and ½ ounce each ginger root and licorice root. Simmer down to 1 quart and strain. Take in wineglassful doses every 2 hours.

Devil's Claw

Harpagophytum procumbens
Sesame Family
Part Used: Root
Habitat: Southern and eastern Africa, clay, sandy soil and waste areas.

Dosage: 60 grains

- **Do not use during pregnancy or while nursing.**
- Stomach acid reduces effectiveness.
- Do not use with anti-coagulant medicines.
- Antibiotics reduce effectiveness during and for two weeks after taking.
- May reduce blood pressure - avoid in presence of congestive heart disease.
- Do not use in presence of ulcers.

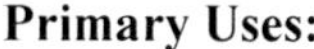

Primary Uses:
Anti-inflammatory
Arthritis
Carpal Tunnel Syndrome, pain
Gout, pain
Pain, especially lower back
Rheumatism
Tendonitis, pain

Secondary Uses:
Appetite stimulant - tea
Digestive problems - tea, soothes
Diuretic
Heartburn - tea
High blood pressure
High blood sugar
Indigestion - tea

External Uses:
Skin disease

- This is a wonderful herb for joint pain. People have had great success in arthritic conditions as well as sports injuries.

Dong Quai

Angelica sinensis
Parsley Family
Part Used: Root
Habitat: China; Japan; Korea.

Also known as: Chinese Angelica Root; Female Ginseng; Tang-kuei

Dosage: 3 - 15 grams

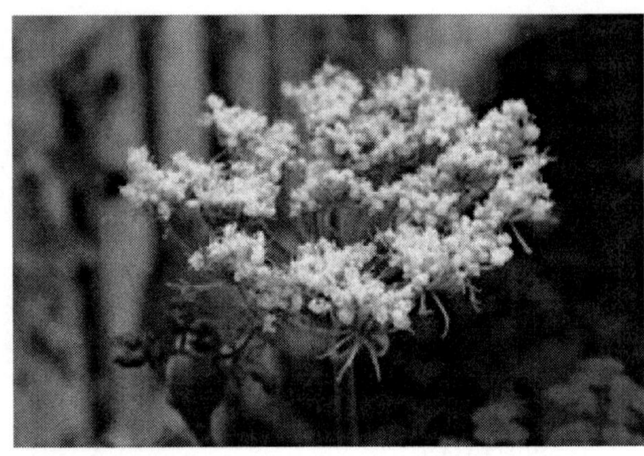

- **Do not use during pregnancy or while nursing.**
- May cause photosensitivity - avoid sunlight while taking.
- Avoid with prescription blood thinners.
- Avoid taking for 30 days after first symptoms of a herpes infection or recurrence - it inhibits the body's defense against the virus.
- Large doses may kill healthy skin cells.

Primary Uses:
Cramps
Hot flashes
Menopause
Menstrual irregularity
Premenstrual Syndrome
Vaginal dryness

Secondary Uses:
Anemia
Blood clots - dissolves
Constipation
High blood pressure, male & female
Insomnia
Liver

Other Possible Uses:
Tonic

- Dong Quai is one of the best herbs to take for all the problems associated with menopause.
- Tinctures decrease menstrual flow and relax the uterus.

Dragon's Blood

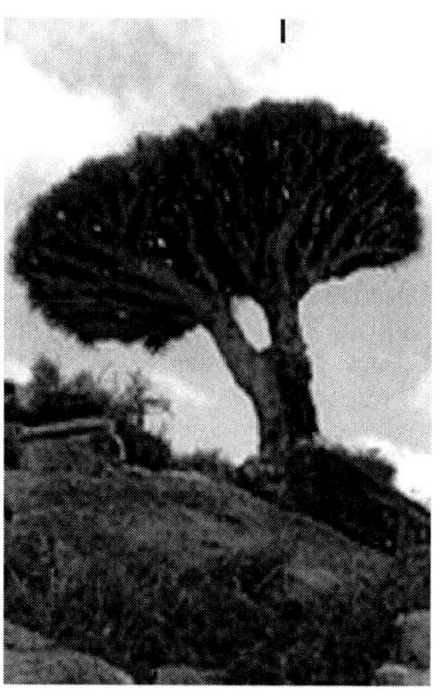

Daemomorops Draco
Palm Family
Part Used: Resin from fruit
Habitat: Sumatra.

Also known as: Blood; Blume; Calamus Draco; Draconis Resina; Dragon's Blood Palm; Dragonis Resina; Sanguis Draconis

Dosage: 10 - 30 grains

- Presently thought to be inert.

Other Possible Uses:
Aphrodisiac
Astringent
Diarrhea
Syphilis

External Uses:
Gleet - douche
Wounds

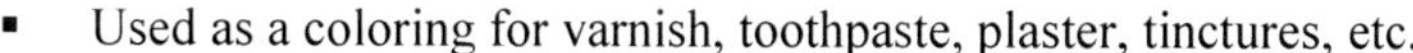

- Used as a coloring for varnish, toothpaste, plaster, tinctures, etc.
- Many people use this solely as an incense.

Echinacea

Echinacea angustifolia; Echinacea purpurea
Composite Family
Parts Used: Leaves, Root
Habitat: America (west of Ohio); Britain.

Also known as: Black Sampson; Coneflower; Purple Coneflower; Rudbeckia

Dosage: 15 - 30 grains

- Do not use if allergic to sunflowers, ragweed or any of the daisy family.
- Do not take more than two weeks at a time. The body builds up resistance to the herb.
- Avoid immediately before, during and after any organ transplant if Neoral, Sandimmune or Prognof are prescribed to prevent rejection of organ.
- Increases T-cells so avoid in the presence of any chronic infection or autoimmune disorder such as Lupus, Multiple Sclerosis, Rheumatoid arthritis, Tuberculosis, HIV or AIDS.
- Do not use if attempting pregnancy - may decrease a woman's fertility and interfere with the release of eggs.

Primary Uses:
Antibiotic
Anti-inflammatory
Antiseptic, blood
Anti-viral
Aphrodisiac
Cancer, colorectal, liver (advanced) - stabilizes white blood cells when having chemotherapy or radiation treatments
Colds
Colic
Detox
Flu
Gonorrhea
Immune function - restores
Infections, all
Lymphatic system
Snakebites
Syphilis

Secondary Uses:
Chronic Fatigue Syndrome
Glandular swelling
Herpes - extract
Lyme disease
Sore throat
Strep throat - preventative
Yeast infections

External Uses:
Acne - cream
Boils
Ear infection (with goldenseal) - heals & stops drainage
Eczema
Fungal infections, nails - cream
Hemorrhoids - enema
Skin wounds
Snakebites
Sore throat - gargle
Sun damage - cream
Toothache
Wounds

- **Seek professional medical attention for snakebites.** Herbs may help, but are not as likely to save a life as our modern techniques regarding poisons.

- Increases production of interferons, which help against colds and flu. Also activates macrophages that help destroy bacteria, viruses and other infections, as well as cancer cells.
- Use a blend for best results – each one is used for specific disorders.

Elder

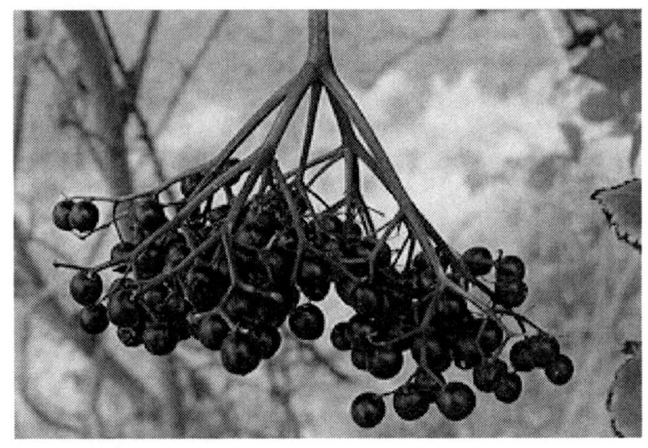

Sambucus nigra
Honeysuckle Family
Parts Used: Bark, Leaves, Flowers, Berries
Habitat: Europe; temperate areas of the world.

Also known as: Alhuren; Bat Tree; Black Elder; Bore Tree; Bour Tree; Boure Tree; Common Elder; Eldrum; Ellhorn; Hollunder; Hylantree; Hylder; Lady Ellhorn; Old Gal; Old Lady; Pipe Tree; Rob Elder; Sureau; Sweet Elder; Tree of Doom

- Uncooked seeds are toxic. Do not eat raw or unripe berries - causes nausea, vomiting and diarrhea.
- Do not use stems - they contain cyanide and can be toxic.
- Roots and leaves may cause diarrhea, nausea and vomiting.
- Large doses of elderberry juice cause uncontrollable diarrhea.

Bark:
Dosage: 30 grains

Primary Uses:
Purgative - strong, infusion 1 ounce to 1 pint

Secondary Uses:
Emetic - larger doses, infusion

Other Possible Uses:
Diuretic
Epilepsy

Leaves:
Dosage: 60 grains

Primary Uses:
Perspiration - produces

Secondary Uses:
Detox
Diuretic
Emetic
Purgative

Other Possible Uses:
Dropsy
Expectorant

External Uses:
Bruises - ointment
Chilblains - ointment
Eye inflammation - tea wash
Inflammation - soothes, ointment
Piles - boiled with linseed oil
Sprains - ointment
Wounds - ointment

Berries:
Dosage: 30 - 60 grains

Primary Uses:
Bronchitis
Colds
Diuretic
Fever - wine, promotes perspiration
Flu - wine, hot at night, promotes perspiration
Laxative - mild
Perspiration - promotes - wine

Secondary Uses:
Asthma - hot wine
Coughs
Emetic - mild

Other Possible Uses:
Colic
Diarrhea
Epilepsy
Piles
Rheumatism
Syphilis

External Uses:
Eczema

Flowers:
Dosage: 30 - 60 grains

Primary Uses:
Astringent – elderflower water
Colds - hot tea at bedtime
Flu - strong infusion with peppermint at bedtime, produces perspiration & sleep (quick cure)
Perspiration - produces, tea

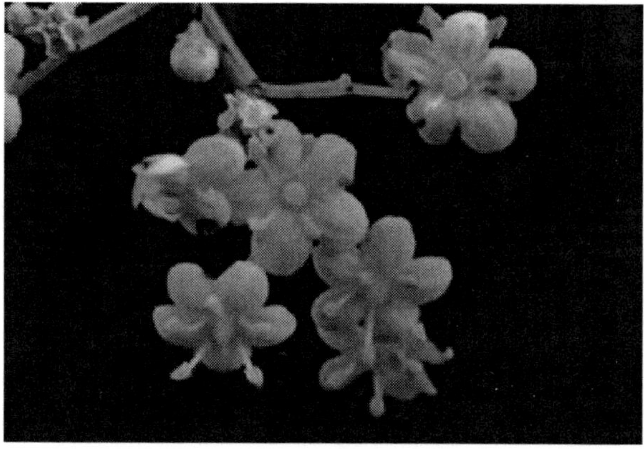

Secondary Uses:
Detox
Laxative - gentle, tea
Stimulant - gentle, elderflower water
Throat problems - hot tea at bedtime

Other Possible Uses:
Bronchitis
Coughs - tea
Pleurisy - tea
Scarlet Fever

External Uses:
Blemishes - water
Boils - water
Burns - ointment
Eyes, inflamed - cold tea
Freckles - water
Hands, chapped - ointment
Headache - water on temples
Hemorrhoids - with honeysuckle in water or milk
Inflammation
Pain
Skin - softens & whitens, bath
Sunburn - water
Tumors - water
Wounds - ointment

- Oil of Elder: Absorb 1 part bruised leaves in 3 parts linseed oil.
- Ointment: 3 parts fresh leaves, 4 parts lard, 2 parts prepared suet. Heat until clear. Strain through linen cloth, apply pressure and cool.
- Ointment #2: ½ pound elder leaves, ¼ pound plantain leaves, 2 ounces ground ivy, 4 ounces green wormwood. Cut into small pieces and boil in 4 pounds of lard over low fire.

Stir continually until leaves are crisp. Strain, then press out ointment.

- Insect repellent: Sprinkle bruised leaves or a decoction on plants.
- Black hair dye: Boil berries in wine.
- Elderflower water: Fill large jar with blossoms. (No stems!) Press. Pour 2 quarts boiling water on them and cool. Add 1-½ ounces spirits. Cover with cloth and keep in a warm place for a few hours. Chill and strain through muslin. Bottle and cork.
- For wine, use English elder. Other elders are too bitter.
- Sambucal is a patented form of this herb, which negates the risk of poisoning by raw or unripe berries.

Elecampane

Inula Helenium
Composite Family
Part Used: Dried Root
Habitat: England; Scotland; pastures and shady places.

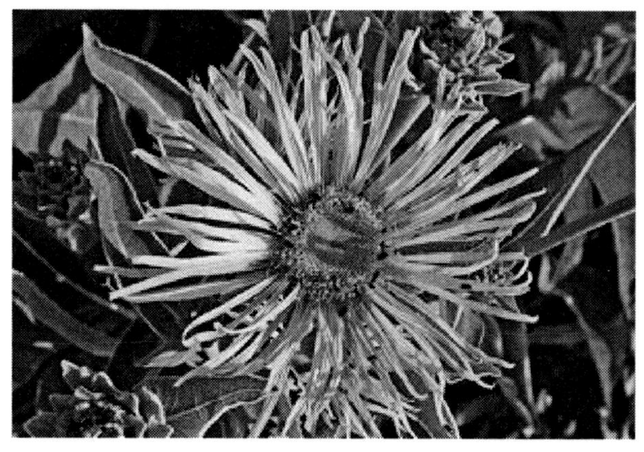

Also known as: Alycompaine; Elf Dock; Horseheal; Inula; Nurse Heal; Scabwort; Sunflower; Velvet Dock; Wild Sunflower

Dosage: 20 - 60 grains

- Repeated use may cause allergic sensitivity.
- Large doses produce cramps, diarrhea and vomiting.
- **Do not use during pregnancy or while nursing.**

Primary Uses:
Asthma
Bronchitis - very good cure
Coughs
Diuretic
Expectorant
Lungs, chronic diseases
Stimulant - gentle
Whooping cough
Tuberculosis
Tonic

Other Possible Uses:
Antiseptic
Astringent
Bactericide - essential oil
Dropsy
Dyspepsia (indigestion)

Secondary Uses:
Congestive heart failure - relieves pain
Detox
Perspiration - produces
Pneumonia
Shortness of breath (upon exertion) - relieves

External Uses:
Antiseptic - used in Spain for surgery
Circulation - increases & produces red skin
Insects - repels (burn)
Sciatica
Skin affections & diseases

- The root makes a great blue dye.
- Dug in autumn, cut up and dried at a high temperature.
- Coats the lining of bronchial passages and stimulates coughing that expels mucous from the lungs.
- The freshly dug root may be hung up as flypaper.

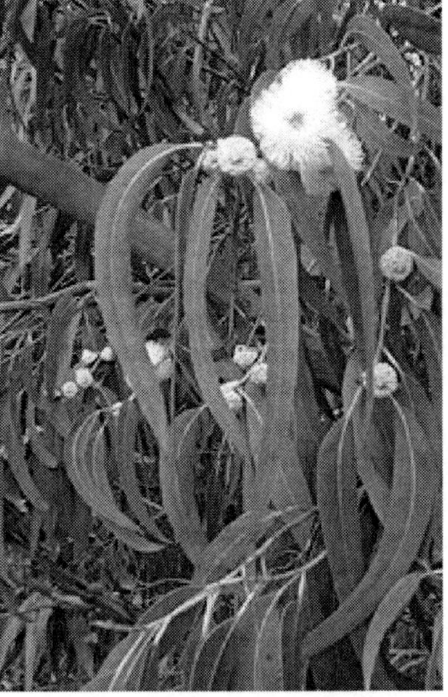

Eucalyptus

Eucalyptus globulus
Clove Family
Part Used: Leaves (oil)
Habitat: Africa; Australia; India; southern Europe.

Also known as: Blue Gum; Cultivated Lucern; Purple Medicle; Red Gum; Stringy Bark Tree

Dosage: 10 - 30 grains

- Do not use in presence of high blood pressure, heart disease, diabetes or thyroid disease.
- Do not overdose.
- Best kept external. May cause respiratory arrest and seizures.
- Do not use on open wounds.
- **Do not use during pregnancy**.
- Some people are allergic and develop an irritating (but harmless) rash.
- Undiluted oil produces serious reactions such as drop in blood pressure, circulation problems, collapse, suffocation and death.
- Do not apply oil to an infant or small child's face, especially near the nose - may cause asthma-like reactions and possible asphyxiation.
- Do not use if have digestive problems, inflammation of the stomach or intestines, a biliary duct disorder or liver disease.
- Never apply oil directly to nostrils.
- Do not use around children with seizure disorders or who have ever had a seizure.
- Do not use on children under two years old for any reason.

Primary Uses:
Cardiac action - increases
Distemper, dogs
Stimulant

External Uses:
Allergies
Antiseptic
Arthritis
Colds & flu - inhale steam from boiling leaves (keep eyes shut)
Cuts, minor - ointment
Decongestant - inhale steam from boiling leaves
Disinfectant
Dust mites - kills, oil
Fleas - repels and kills, oil
Headache (tension) - oil, rubbed on temples
Insect bites - ointment
Muscle soreness - ointment
Pain
Parasitic skin infections
Sinusitis

- The oil may be combined with equal parts of pennyroyal oil and sprayed in hen houses and runs to keep ticks away. This mixture also works to rid dogs and cats of fleas when used as a bath. (Do not rinse off.)

Eyebright

Euphrasia officinalis
Snapdragon Family
Parts Used: Aerial (above ground) parts
Habitat: Europe; North America; northern and western Asia.

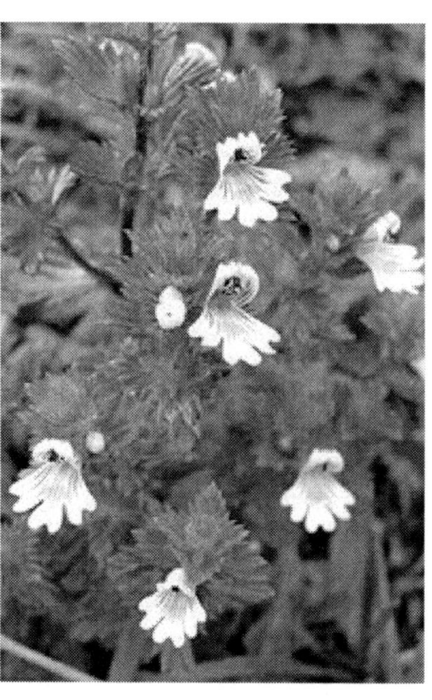

Also known as: Augentrost; Euphorasia; Euphrosyne; Red Eyebright

Dosage: 60 grains

Primary Uses:
Astringent
Eye diseases & weakness
Ophthalmia
Tonic - slight

Other Possible Uses:
Colds
Hay fever
Headache
Memory
Runny nose
Stomachic

External Uses:
Eyes, all disorders - especially with goldenseal (use fresh juice or infuse in milk or water) 1 ounce to 1 pint, bathe eyes 3-4x a day. (warm)
Eyes, inflammation, pain, allergies & itchy
Eyestrain
Ophthalmia
Very good for irritated eyes due to hay fever, taken both internally and externally. (Compresses, eye drops and baths.)

False Unicorn

Chamaelirium luteum
Lily Family
Part Used: Root
Habitat: East of the Mississippi, low moist ground.

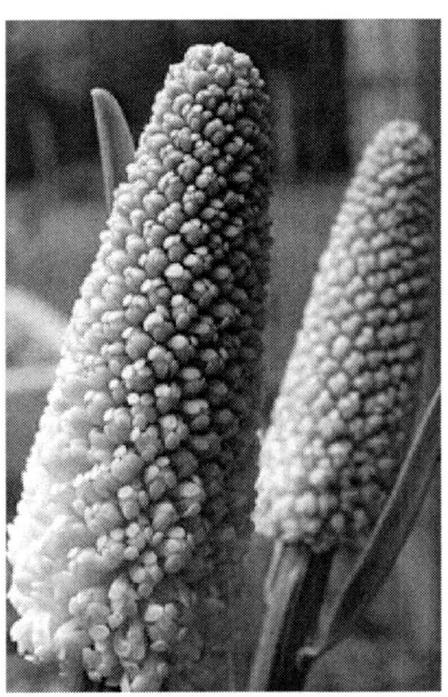

Also known as: Helonias; Helonias Dioica; Helonias Lutea; Starwort; Veratrum Luteum

Dosage: 15 - 30 grains

- **In large doses it is a cardiac poison.**

Primary Uses:
Female disorders
Menstrual pain
Premenstrual Syndrome

Secondary Uses:
Diuretic
Impotence
Infertility
Prostate disorders
Tonic
Worms

Other Possible Uses:
Detox
Emetic
Kidney diseases
Liver diseases
Urinary irritability & weakness

Fennel

Foeniculum vulgare
Parsley Family
Parts Used: Seeds, Leaves, Roots
Habitat: Mediterranean shores to India; temperate Europe; on limestone soils, dry soils and near seacoasts.

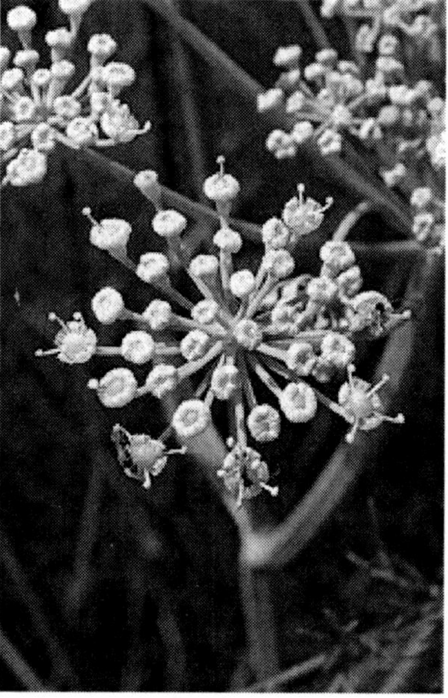

Also known as: Fenkel; Sweet Fennel; Wild Fennel

Dosage: 15 - 30 grains

- Fennel oil causes nausea and breathing problems.
- Interferes with Cipro.
- May have possible contradictory effects on the liver - avoid in the presence of hepatitis, alcoholism or liver disease. (Unconfirmed.)
- Has a sugar content - use with caution with diabetes.
- Increases concentration of estrogen in bloodstream.
- Avoid large quantities during pregnancy or in presence of an estrogen disorder such as breast or uterine cancer, fibroids, ovarian cysts, etc.

Primary Uses:
Asthma
Bronchitis
Cough - syrup with honey
Diuretic - tea, safe
Emmenagogue
Gas - tea (especially in children), 1 tsp. to 1 cup water or milk (one of the best & safest)
Hiccups - tea
Indigestion
Milk - stimulates
Motion sickness
Nausea - tea
Obesity - tea
Purgative - gentle
Stones, all
Vomiting

Secondary Uses:
Antimicrobial
Appetite stimulant
Colic
Crohn's disease
Digestion - soothes
Fever
Food poisoning - kills some types of bacteria
Gout
Jaundice
Hernia - heals
Liver
Muscle strain - heals
Poison from vegetables (mushrooms & herbs) - boiled in wine
Spleen
Wheezing

External Uses:
Arthritis - oil
Conjunctivitis - compress
Dermatitis - compress
Eyes, tired & sore - fennel water
Fleas - on ground, around kennels, etc.
Rheumatism – oil

- Fennel is used in scenting soaps and perfumes.
- Compress is made from the tea. Also available in health food stores are lozenges, honeys, juices, syrups, water and tea.
- If no improvement is noticed after using for 2 weeks, check for a possible misdiagnosis of the disorder being treated.
- Tea is great for nursing mothers for milk production and to help infants with breathing problems.

Fenugreek

Trigonella Foenum-graecum
Legume Family
Part Used: Seeds
Habitat: Africa; eastern shores of the Mediterranean; Egypt; England; India; Morocco.

Also known as: Bird's Foot; Greek Hay-Seed

Dosage: 60 grains

- **Do not use during pregnancy**.
- May interfere with iron absorption - do not use in presence of anemia.
- May interfere with thyroid hormones.
- Large doses (100 grams) produce intestinal upset and nausea.
- May enhance the effect of insulin or blood sugar lowering medications and lower blood sugar too far.

Primary Uses:
Anemia
Diabetes - may be used with insulin
Fever - reduces - soak seeds in water until they form a thick paste
Gout
Lungs
Stomach

Secondary Uses:
Asthma
Expectorant
Laxative
Mastitis - promotes lactation & eases symptoms
Sinusitis

Other Possible Uses:
Blood sugar - lowers

External Uses:
Abscesses - poultice
Boils - poultice
Inflammation - ointment
Sore throat – gargle

- Soak seeds in warm water until they form a thick paste to make ointments, gruel, etc.
- Coats the lining of the intestines, keeps the stomach from emptying quickly and makes glucose enter the bloodstream more slowly after meals.
- Stimulates the pancreas to secrete insulin and helps the liver and muscle tissue respond better to insulin.
- Reduces excretion of glucose in urine.
- Helps lower LDL levels without affecting HDL levels.
- Stimulates the growth of breast tissue due to the change in liver enzymes that slow the rate at which a woman's body breaks down estrogen.

Feverfew

Chrysanthemum Parthenium
Composite Family
Parts Used: Aerial Parts
Habitat: Australia; Europe; North America.

Also known as: Bachelor's Buttons; Featherfew; Febrifuge Plant

Dosage: 30 - 60 grains

- Chewing on the fresh leaves may cause mouth ulcers - discontinue if ulcers develop.
- Skin contact with the fresh plant may cause rash, especially if sensitive to ragweed, marigold, chrysanthemums, daisies, sunflowers, chamomile or asters.
- Use with caution if allergic to ragweed.
- Do not use with blood thinners or for 2 weeks prior to any surgery.
- **Do not use during pregnancy** - may cause uterine contractions and bleeding.

Primary Uses:
Arthritis
Colds
Coughs - with honey
Depression
Emmenagogue
Fever
Gas
Headache
Hysteria
Indigestion
Migraines - one of the best*
Muscle tension
Nerves
Wheezing - with honey
Worms - expels

Secondary Uses:
Lupus
Rheumatoid arthritis, pain - take 3 months+

Other Possible Uses:
Dizziness
Opium overdose - remedy**
Stimulant

External Uses:
Insect bites – tincture

* Produces serotonin (must use for 4 months minimum). Also reduces vomiting and visual distortion. May not reduce the duration of an attack, but does lessen frequency and severity.
**As with any overdose - seek the help of a hospital or doctor, as the herbal remedies are not as capable as modern medicine for this type of problem.

- Does not cause stomach upset or constipation.
- For migraines - must be taken on a daily basis with no exception. It may take two months or more for it to penetrate the system and stop migraines from occurring.

Frankincense

Boswellia Thurifera
Frankincense Family
Part Used: Gum Resin
Habitat: Arabia; Somaliland.

Also known as: Incense; Olibans; Olibanum; Olibanus

Dosage: 3 - 10 grams

Primary Uses:
Antidote, hemlock
Laryngitis
Leprosy (used in China)
Stimulant
Tumors

Secondary Uses:
Dysentery
Fever
Nerves
Ulcers
Vomiting

External Uses:
Aromatic
Astringent
Gonorrhea
Wounds, abnormal mucus discharge

Garlic

Allium sativum
Lily Family
Part Used: Bulb
Habitat: Worldwide.

Also known as: Poor Man's Treacle; Stinkweed

Dosage: 2 - 3 cloves

- **Do not use when nursing - may pass through milk and cause colic.**
- Do not eat more than ten cloves per day.
- Do not use with blood thinners - may intensify effect of anticoagulants or antihypertensives.
- May interfere with medication for lowering blood sugar.
- Avoid for 2 weeks prior to surgery due to increased risk of bleeding.
- May cause heartburn and gas

Primary Uses:
Antibiotic
Anti-fungal
Anti-parasitic
Antiseptic
Antiviral
Arthritis
Asthma - syrup
Blood clots - reduce
Bronchitis - syrup
Cancer*
Circulation
Colds
Coughs - syrup
Detox
Diuretic
Expectorant
Flu
Heart attack, prevents
High blood pressure
High cholesterol
Hoarseness - syrup
Indigestion
Infection, all
Insomnia
Leprosy
Liver disease
Perspiration - produces
Stimulant
Stroke - prevents
Ulcers, peptic - inhibits growth of Helicobacter pylori
Yeast infection

Secondary Uses:
Antibacterial
Bladder infection
Diabetes**
Diarrhea
Gas
Heart disease - prevents
Sinuses
Strep throat
Tumors
Vaginitis
Yeast infections - inhibits Candida Albicans

Other Possible Uses:
Abscesses
Catarrh
Hysteria
Infantile catarrh
Intestinal complaints
Lungs
Ringworm
Saliva - produces
Tuberculosis

External Uses:
Antiseptic
Ear infection - oil applied directly to ear canal
Gangrene - preventative

Inhibits fungus, mold & yeast
Insect bites
Mosquitoes - kills larvae in ponds
Snakebites
Tumors
Warts
Wounds – disinfects

*May help with chemotherapy by reducing the production of free radicals, but may increase bleeding. Boosts antibiotics and works well with cancer treatments. Reduces production of free radicals in liver and lung tissue, and inhibits the growth of Helicobacter pylori, one of the factors of stomach cancer. May lower rate of breast, colon, larynx and stomach cancer in both men and women, esophageal in men. Slows breast and prostate cancer cells. Prevents tumors from developing their own blood supplies, stops their formation after carcinogenic chemicals and inhibits the speed of tumors once they have begun.

**Lowers triglycerides in blood, ties up receptors that deactivate insulin and stimulates the pancreas to secrete insulin. Inhibits platelet stickiness, slowing blood coagulation.

- Syrup: One quart of boiling water poured on one pound of fresh root cut into slices. Put in an enclosed vessel for 12 hours. Add honey to make syrup. You may add boiled fresh fennel to cover odor.
- Simmer garlic with cabbage to cut down on the odor. Add honey to taste. Adults may drink this freely.
- 3 or 4 crushed garlic heads added to bran or molasses mix will worm a horse of 14 to 15 hands. 1 clove added to fish oil may be fed to cats to worm them. 2 cloves in fish oil for medium to large dogs.

Ginger

Zingiber officinale
Ginger Family
Part Used: Root
Habitat: Africa; Asia; Jamaica; West Indies.

Also known as: African Ginger; Jamaica Ginger

Dosage: 10 grains

- Use caution with sleeping aids - may prolong sleep when used with barbiturates as well as increase their absorption in the digestive tract.
- Avoid essence of ginger - it is often adulterated with harmful ingredients.
- Do not use in presence of gallstones - increases bile flow.
- Increases potency of blood clot preventatives and may result in unexpected bleeding. Stop taking 4 days prior to surgery - makes blood platelets less sticky and increases risk of bleeding. May be taken immediately after surgery as long as bleeding is not a risk.
- May interfere with iron and fat-soluble vitamin absorption.
- Large doses may stimulate uterine contractions. Ginger tea is ok up to 10 cups a day during pregnancy.

Primary Uses:
Alcoholic gastritis
Appetite stimulant
Cancer, nausea from chemotherapy
Circulation - stimulant
Colic
Colitis
Constipation, cramping
Diarrhea
Digestion
Gas
Indigestion
Motion sickness - one of the best
Morning sickness - 1st two months only
Nausea (even after surgery)
Pain, stomach
Perspiration - produces
Stimulant
Vomiting (even after surgery)

Secondary Uses:
Allergies, food & environmental
Anti-inflammatory
Arthritis
Asthma
Colds - tea
Cramps
Dysentery
Fever
Flu
High cholesterol - slows liver production
Hot flashes
Infection, parasitic*
Pain
Spasms
Strep throat
Ulcers, peptic

Other Possible Uses:
Anticonvulsant
Antispasmodic
Aphrodisiac
Astringent
Cold hands and feet
Expectorant
Headache

External Uses:
Burns, minor - compress
Dandruff - with olive oil
Earache - warm oil
Hair growth - tea
Inflammation – compress

* Dissolves parasites and their eggs, making it wonderful for use with sushi since it kills the

Anisakid worm within 16 hours, which is sometimes carried in raw fish. The tea is good for schistosomiasis, a parasitic disease increasingly prevalent in tourists returning to the United States.

- Used in China as a tea to turn breech babies (before delivery).
- Take with plenty of water to avoid the burning sensation it may produce in the throat. If using with chemotherapy, take with food to reduce stomach irritation.
- Ginger ale: Simmer a 3 or 4-inch piece of ginger root in 2-½ cups water for 20 minutes. Strain, cool and refrigerate. Add carbonated water and honey to taste.
- Ginger beer: Pour 5 quarts water over 1 sliced lemon, 1 ounce chopped ginger and 2 cups sugar. Stir until sugar is dissolved. Spread ½ ounce fresh yeast onto a slice of toast and add to the lukewarm liquid. Stand for 12 hours in a warm place. Strain and bottle. Place in a cool place. Will be ready to drink in one week.

Gingko Biloba

Gingko biloba
Gingko Family
Part Used: Leaves
Habitat: China; eastern United States; France; Japan.

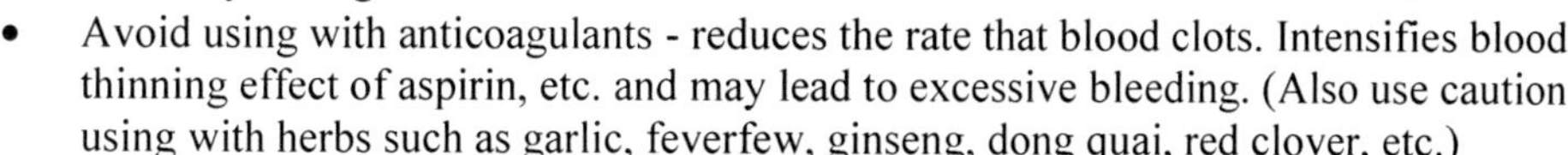

Also known as: Maidenhair Tree

Dosage: 240 mg per day maximum

- Large doses over a period of time may damage liver.
- Avoid using with anticoagulants - reduces the rate that blood clots. Intensifies blood thinning effect of aspirin, etc. and may lead to excessive bleeding. (Also use caution using with herbs such as garlic, feverfew, ginseng, dong quai, red clover, etc.)
- May increase blood pressure when combined with Thiazide diuretics for high blood pressure.
- Affects insulin secretion and altars blood glucose levels.
- High doses produce disorientation and intoxication.
- May cause headache, irritability, restlessness, diarrhea, nausea, vomiting, palpitations, weakness, skin rash, dizziness and vertigo. These are usually weak and transient.
- Unprocessed leaves may trigger allergic reactions - use extreme caution (even in teas).
- May interact with monoamine oxidase inhibitors and increase risk of seizure.

Primary Uses:
Alzheimer's, symptoms
Antioxidant
Brain function
Circulation, all, especially brain
Concentration
Dizziness
Ears, ringing, hearing loss
Impotence - increases blood supply
Leg cramps, due to circulation
Memory loss
Oxygen, brain

Secondary Uses:
Attention Deficit Disorder, adult
Allergies, inflammation
Asthma
Cancer - prevents tumors from developing a blood supply*
Coughs
Diabetic retinopathy
Expectorant
Hearing
Heart disorders
Kidney disorders
Multiple Sclerosis - prevents relapse
Parkinson's disease
Phlebitis
Stroke
Vertigo
Vision - increases circulation & prevents destruction of ocular nerve in glaucoma

Other Possible Uses:
Depression
Eczema
Headaches
Senility

External Uses:
Hemorrhoids

* Tea slows growth of colon, lung and liver cancers, helps kill leukemia and lymphoma cells, and inhibits growth of bladder, breast and possible ovarian cancers.

- Inhibits development of plaque in blood and scavenges free radicals in the brain and spine.

Golden Seal

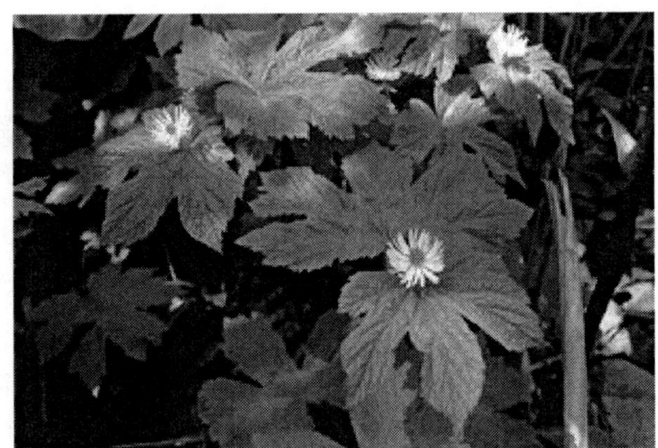

Hydrastis Canadensis
Buttercup Family
Part Used: Root from a 3-year-old plant, dried in open air
Habitat: Canada; eastern United States; shady woods and moist areas at edges of woods.

Also known as: Eye Balm; Eye Root; Ground Raspberry; Indian Dye; Indian Paint; Jaundice Root; Orange Root; Turmeric Root; Warnera; Wild Curcuma; Yellow Puccoon; Yellow Root

Dosage: 30 grains; 1 tsp. to 1 pint hot water

- **Do not use during pregnancy - abortive.**
- **Do not use while nursing.**
- Do not use for more than two consecutive weeks - may become toxic in body. Take a 2 week break in between each usage.
- Do not use in presence of high blood pressure, heart disease, diabetes or glaucoma.
- Do not use if allergic to ragweed.
- Large doses irritate mucous membranes in the mouth, cause diarrhea, nausea, vomiting, slowed heart rate and respiratory problems.
- May limit effectiveness of the anticoagulants Heparin and Warfarin (Coumadin).
- May interfere with absorption of Tetracycline.
- May lower blood sugar levels.

Primary Uses:
Antibacterial
Antibiotic
Anti-inflammatory
Appetite stimulant
Bowels, catarrh
Colds
Colon, chronic inflammation
Constipation, habitual
Detox
Diabetes - increases effectiveness of insulin
Digestion
Flu
Gas
Glandular swelling
Heartburn, from emotional tension
High blood pressure
Hypoglycemia - be careful, increases insulin
Immune system function
Infections
Insulin - potentiates
Laxative
Liver problems
Lymphatic system
Morning sickness
Mucus membranes, inflamed
Nausea
Pancreas
Sinus
Spleen
Stomach problems
Tonic
Ulcers, peptic with myrrh (half & half)
Vomiting

Secondary Uses:
Alcoholism - with cayenne
Inflammation
Muscular tissues
Pain

Other Possible Uses:
Anticonvulsive, intestines
Bronchitis
Staphylococcus

External Uses:
Acne
Boils
Canker sores - wash
Eczema
Eyes, sore - wash
Fungal infections - douche
Gonorrhea
Hemorrhoids - enema
Mouth sores
Periodontal disease - destroys the bacteria that causes inflamed gums
Ringworm - tea, rub
Syphilis
Ulcers
Wounds

- Douche: Dissolve 1 tbls. powder in warm water and let cool. Use every 3 days for up to 2 weeks.
- Take with meals for best results.
- Put extract on cotton and pack tightly between lips and gums for mouth pain.

Gotu Kola

Centella Asiatica
Parsley Family
Part Used: Leaves
Habitat: Africa, Australia; India; South America; southern United States.

Also known as: Centella; Indian Pennywort

Dosage: 200 - 800 mg per day

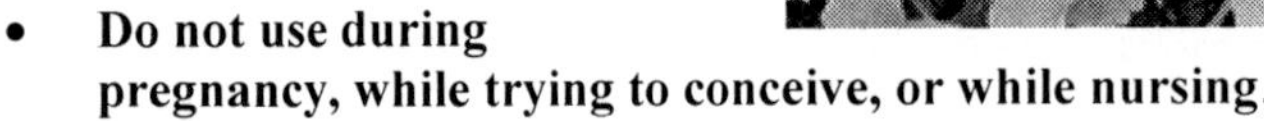

- **Do not use during pregnancy, while trying to conceive, or while nursing**.
- If nausea develops, lower the dosage.
- May interfere with oral diabetes medications.
- May raise cholesterol levels.
- Do not take with niacin.
- May have a narcotic effect - do not take with tranquilizers.
- Do not give to children under 2 years old.

Primary Uses:
Aphrodisiac
Appetite stimulant
Blood diseases
Childbirth - promotes healing after
Circulation
Congestive heart failure
Depression
Diuretic
Fatigue
Fever
Hepatitis
High blood pressure
Insomnia
Kidney stones
Liver function, especially alcoholic
Measles
Mental disorders
Nerve tonic
Rheumatism
Sore throat
Stress
Tissues - shrinks
Tonsillitis
Urinary tract infections
Venereal diseases

Secondary Uses:
Alzheimer's
Ankles, swollen
Cellulite
Congestion
Episiotomy - heals
Leg cramps
Leg swelling
Memory enhancement
Phlebitis
Varicose veins

Other Possible Uses:
Leprosy
Rejuvenative
Relaxant
Restorative

External Uses:
Burns
Episiotomy - heals
Psoriasis
Scarring
Wounds

- Great for bed-ridden people. It increases blood flow and promotes healing.
- Sometimes served as a salad or cooked vegetable in India.
- Use the cream externally to stimulate cell regeneration.
- Increases oxygen to veins, decreases carbon dioxide to muscles and stabilizes connective tissue around veins.

Gravel Root

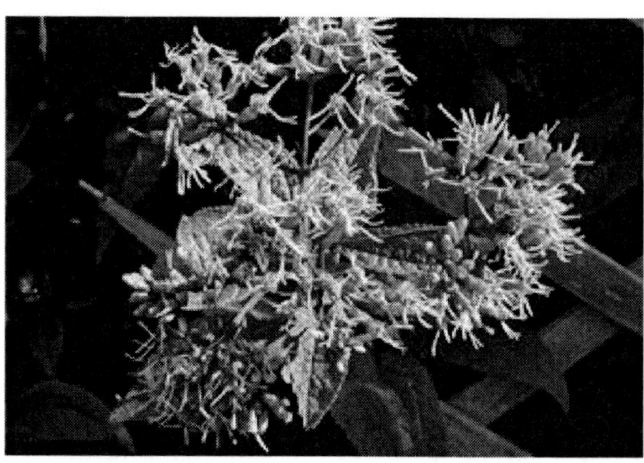

Eupatorium purpureum
Composite Family
Part Used: Fresh Root
Habitat: Canada; North America; swampy low grounds.

Also known as: Gravelweed; Hempweed; Joe-Pye Weed; Jopi Weed; Purple Boneset; Queen of the Meadow Root; Trumpet-Weed

Dosage: 30 grains

Primary Uses:
Astringent
Diuretic
Dropsy
Gout
Nervine
Rheumatism
Stimulant

Secondary Uses:
Endometriosis
Kidneys, infections & stones
Labor pains
Leucorrhoea
Menstrual pain
Pelvic inflammatory disease
Prostate inflammation
Urinary infections & stones

Green Tea

Camellia sinensis
Tea Family
Part Used: Dried Leaves & Buds
Habitat: China; India; Sri Lanka.

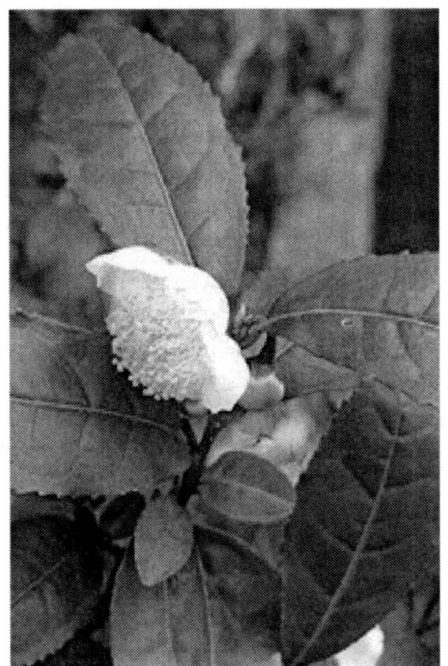

Also known as: Matcha

Dosage: 3 cups of tea per day minimum or 240-320 mg

- **Do not use during pregnancy or while nursing.**
- Do not use in presence of diabetes.
- Do not use in presence of flu. Only use as a preventative.
- Do not take within 1 hour of other medications.
- Do not use with ginseng - reduces the effectiveness of ginseng.
- Do not use in presence of monoamine oxidase inhibitors or blood thinners - negates them due to the levels of vitamin K.

Primary Uses:
Antioxidant
Arteriosclerosis
Asthma - relaxes bronchial tubes
Bronchitis
Cancer*
Cirrhosis - protects from free radicals
Diabetes - suppresses the formation of sticky blood proteins & keeps sugar out of the bloodstream by inhibiting the breakdown of carbs into simple sugars
Endometriosis
Flu - prevents viruses from replicating.
Food poisoning - kills food-borne bacteria,especially Clostridium (which is associated with colon cancer)
High blood pressure
High cholesterol
Mental fatigue
Obesity
Stimulant

External Uses:
Ear infection
Eczema - compress
Herpes - compress, use before Interferon, let dry, then use Interferon
Periodontal disease - prevents dental plaque from forming
Wrinkles - compress

* Green tea has been used for the following types of cancer: colon, skin, esophageal, stomach, breast, ovarian, uterine, pancreatic, lung and small intestine. It blocks cancer-causing compounds and keeps cells from receiving estrogen. Has also been used to prevent development of thyroid cancer from radiation treatments. Protects liver from cancer due to free radicals. Prevents growth of tumors in colorectal cancer.

- Some green tea has caffeine and some do not. If you are concerned, ask before drinking.
- Green tea is known to stain teeth more than coffee, wine or even cigarettes. You may notice your teeth turning a greenish brown, especially between your teeth. Whiteners can help and a good dental cleaning can get rid of the stains.

Guarana

Paullinia Cupana
Soapberry Family
Part Used: Crushed Seeds
Habitat: Brazil; Uruguay.

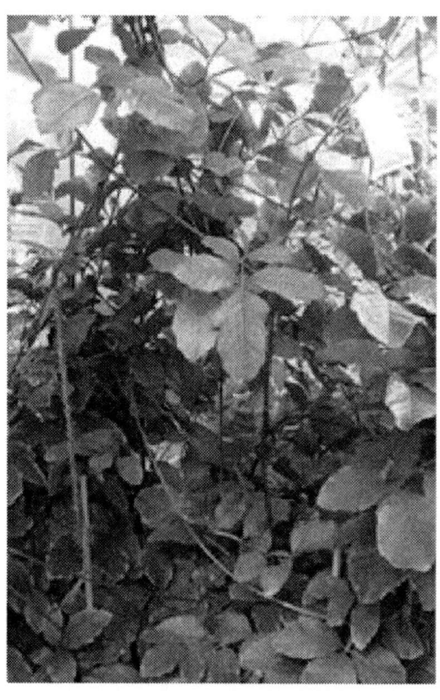

Also known as: Brazilian Cocoa; Guarana Bread; Guarano; Paullinia Sorbilis; Uabano; Uaranazeiro; Wachite

Dosage: 20 - 60 grains

- Contains caffeine.
- Will increase heart rate, possibly also temperature and arterial tension.

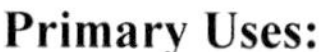

Primary Uses:
Appetite suppressant
Excitant - gentle
Exhaustion
Fatigue
Headache, rheumatic, nervous or menstrual
Stimulant - slightly narcotic

Secondary Uses:
Hangover
Nervine
Tonic

Other Possible Uses:
Aphrodisiac
Diarrhea - mild
Diuretic
Fever - reduces
Leucorrhoea - mild
Urinary infections

Hawthorne

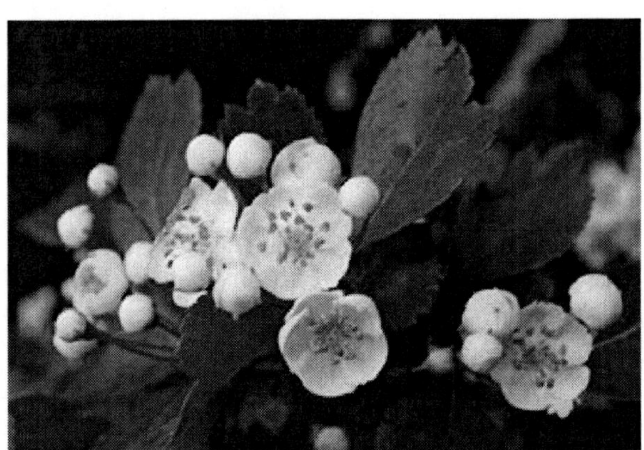

Crataegus oxyacantha
Rose Family
Parts Used: Dried Fruits, Tops, Flowers, Leaves
Habitat: Europe; North America; western Asia.

Also known as: Bread and Cheese Tree; Gaxels; Gazels; Hagthorn; Halves; Haw; Hazels; Huath; Japanese Hawthorne; Ladie's Meat; May; May Blossom, Maybush; May Tree; Quick; Quickset; Thorn; Thorn-Apple Tree; Tree of Chastity; Whitethorn

Dosage: 60 grains

Primary Uses:
Blood vessels - strengthens
Cardiac
Cardiovascular disorders
Circulatory disorders
Coronary blood vessels - dilates
Heart - increases flow of blood & oxygen, flowers & leaves
Heart attack - speeds recovery
Heart muscle - restores, flowers & leaves
High blood pressure - flowers & leaves
High cholesterol
Stroke

Secondary Uses:
Attention Deficit Disorder, children
Ankles, swollen
Arthritis*
Alzheimer's - increases oxygen to brain
Astringent
Cancer, leukemia - accelerates death of leukemia cells
Diuretic
Dropsy
Fractures*
Glaucoma
Halitosis
Kidney troubles - berries
Lupus
Memory loss - increases oxygen to brain
Osteoporosis*
Rheumatism
Varicose veins

Other Possible Uses:
Anemia
Diarrhea
Digestive problems
High blood pressure
Immune system - boosts
Insomnia
Obesity
Sedative - mild
Sore throat
Tonic
External Uses
Acne
Blemishes

*Stabilizes collagen in cartilage and reduces joint damage.

- Dilates blood vessels and helps more oxygen-rich blood get to the heart. Also helps relieve the pain associated with angina pectoris.

Hemlock

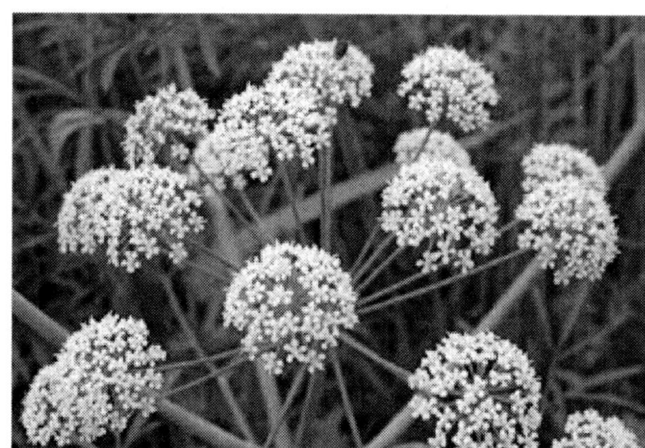

Conium maculatum; Cicuta virosa (Water Hemlock); Circuta maculata
Carrot or Parsley Family
Parts Used: Leaves, Fruit, Seeds
Habitat: Asia; Britain; Europe; North America; South America.

Also known as: Beaver Poison; Herb Bennet; Kecksies; Kex; Musquash Root; Poison Hemlock; Poison Parsley; Spotted Corobane; Spotted Hemlock; Water Parsley

Dosage: 1 - 3 grains

- **POISON! All hemlocks are poisonous.**

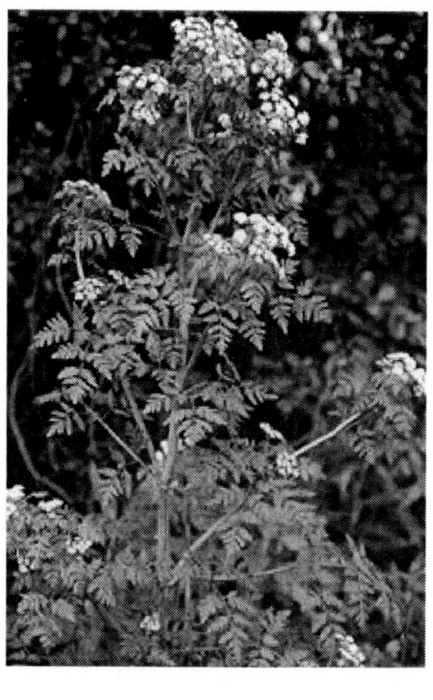

Primary Uses:
Astringent
Pain from ulcers, gout, arthritis
Sedative

Antidotes (for Hemlock Poisoning):
Coffee
Mustard & castor oil emetic
Tannic acid
Zinc emetic
Keep body temperature up!

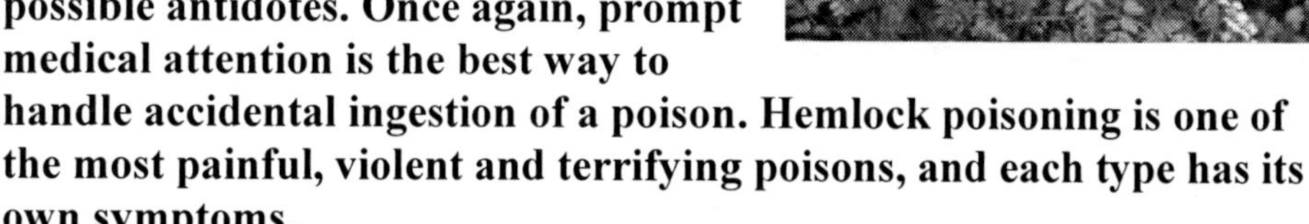

- **Under no circumstances should this herb be used internally as it is extremely poisonous. The reason it is listed in this book is to show the possible antidotes. Once again, prompt medical attention is the best way to handle accidental ingestion of a poison. Hemlock poisoning is one of the most painful, violent and terrifying poisons, and each type has its own symptoms.**
- **Quail love to eat hemlock. It poisons the meat for human consumption though, so be wary of where the quail you consume lives and eats.**

Hemp

Cannabis sativa
Nettle Family
Parts Used: Dried, flowering tops of the female plant
Habitat: India; cultivated worldwide.

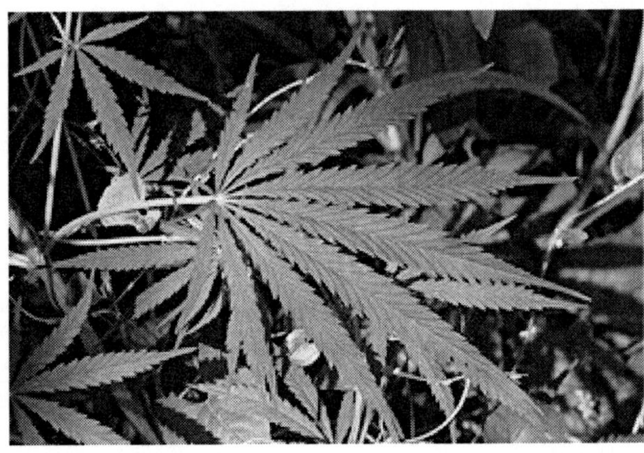

Also known as: Cannabis Chinese; Cannabis Indica; Chanvre; Gallowgrass; Ganeb; Ganja; Hanf; Indian Hemp; Kif; Marijuana; Neckweede; Tekrouri; Weed

Dosage: 1 - 3 grains

- **Poison.**
- Deteriorates rapidly if not in a hermetically sealed container.

Primary Uses:
Antispasmodic
Appetite stimulant
Glaucoma
Gout, pain
Hypnotic
Insomnia
Nervine
Nervous disorders
Neuralgia
Pain
Rheumatism
Sedative

Secondary Uses:
Aphrodisiac
D.T.'s
Depression, mental
Hysteria
Morphine addiction
Stimulant

Other Possible Uses:
Cystitis, chronic - tincture
Delirium
Gonorrhea - tincture (equal parts male & female tops in blossom, bruise & express. 1-3 drops every 2-3 hours)
Infantile convulsions
Insanity
Menorrhagia - tincture
Urinary problems, painful - tincture
Uterus, after pains & prolapsed

Antidote (for overdose):
Coffee
Lemonade - strong
Tannin

- **This herb is illegal in many countries. If you live in or visit a country where it is illegal, find an alternative treatment for the above conditions.**

Henna

Lawsonia alba
Myrtle or Loosestrife Family
Parts Used: Flowers, Powdered Leaves, Fruit
Habitat: Egypt; India; Kurdistan; Levant; Persia; Syria.

Also known as: Al-henna; Al-henne; Al-Khanna; Egyptian Privet; Henne; Hennha; Jamaica Migonette; Mehndi; Mendee; Smooth Lawsonia

Dosage: 60 grains

Primary Uses:
Headache - decoction
Migraine

Secondary Uses:
Leprosy
Smallpox

Other Possible Uses:
Emmenagogue - fruit
Gangrene
Jaundice
Nails, brittle

External Uses:
Gangrene
Leprosy
Skin affections
Smallpox

- Dye for hair, skin & nails - when mixed with the leaves of other plants.

Honeysuckle

Lonicera caprifolium
Honeysuckle Family
Parts Used: Leaves, Flowers, Bark, Seeds
Habitat: Northern temperate zones extending to higher and cool tropical regions.

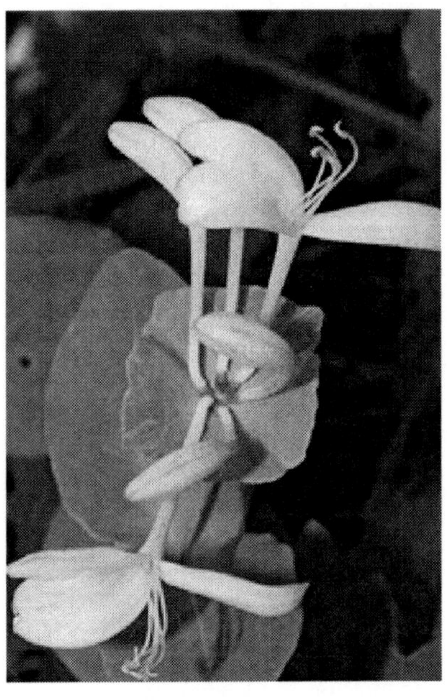

Also known as: Dutch Honeysuckle; Goat's Leaf; Woodbind; Woodbine

Dosage: 10 - 20 grams per day

Primary Uses:
Asthma, nervous - syrup
Lung disorders - syrup of flowers

Secondary Uses:
Diuretic
Hiccups
Increase blood flow to the dermas
Perspiration - produces profuse

Other Possible Uses:
Antispasmodic
Cramps - leaves infused in oil
Headache, nervous - distilled water of
Spleen diseases - syrup of flowers

External Uses:
Eruptions - bark, lotion
Restore circulation to extremities numbed by cold - warm oil
Skin, itchy - bark, lotion
Sore throat - bark, gargle

- Steep flowers in oil set out in the sun.

Hops

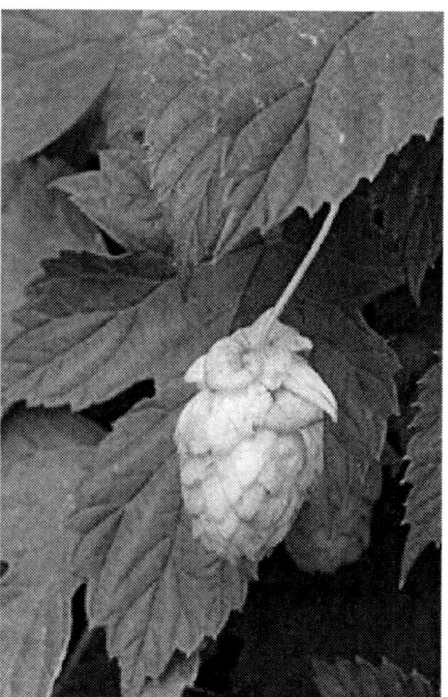

Humulus Lupulus
Nettle Family
Part Used: Flowers of the female plant, aged 2 years
Habitat: Britain; Ireland; Scotland; most northern temperate zones.

Also known as: Beer Flower; Cultivated Lucern; Purple Medicle

Dosage: 30 - 90 grains

- **Do not use during pregnancy.**
- Do not use in presence of an estrogen sensitive disorder such as breast cancer, erectile dysfunction, etc.
- Do not use if trying to lose weight - causes fat deposits around the stomach.
- Avoid 2 weeks prior to surgery - it increases the potency of anesthesia.
- Aggravates depression.
- Do not use with insomnia or anxiety medications.
- Do not give to children before they reach puberty. It contains the most potent of all plant estrogens and is bad for both young boys and girls.
- Do not use with anxiety medications.

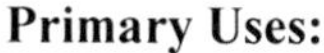

Primary Uses:
Anxiety
Appetite stimulant
Bladder irritation
Brain fatigue & overuse
Delirium
Detox - juice
Diuretic
D.T.'s
Earache
Gonorrhea
Heart disease
Hyperactivity
Hypnotic - with alcohol
Hysteria
Insomnia, due to overwrought brain
Jaundice
Liver problems, sluggish - tea
Muscle cramps
Nervousness
Pain
Restlessness
Sedative
Shock
Stomach problems
Stress
Toothache
Ulcers

Secondary Uses:
Cardiovascular disease
Gas
Indigestion

Other Possible Uses:
Fever
Mother's milk
Poison - expels

External Uses:
Boils - with chamomile
Bruises - with chamomile
Inflammation - with chamomile (one of the best)
Itching
Pain remover - with chamomile
Rheumatism - with chamomile
Sores

- Stimulates the release of bile and makes the stomach secrete digestive fluids, helping digest foods and relieving flatulence.

Horehound

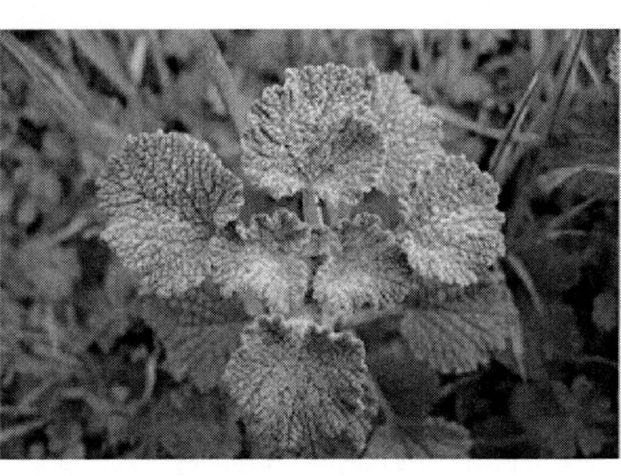

Marrubium vulgare
Mint Family
Parts Used: All Aerial Parts
Habitat: Britain; Europe; in waste places and roadsides.

Also known as: Bull's Blood; Eye of the Star; Hoarhound; Marrubio; Marrubium; Maruil; Marvel; Seed of Horus; Soldier's Tea; White Horehound

Dosage: 15 - 60 grains

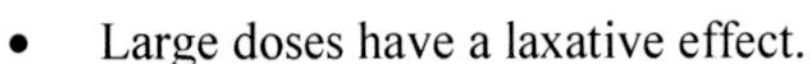

- Large doses have a laxative effect.
- Increases menstrual flow.
- **Do not use during pregnancy or while nursing.**
- Do not give to children under 18 or adults over 65.

Primary Uses:
Asthma
Bronchitis
Colds
Coughs, chronic - syrup
Coughs, smokers with equal parts hyssop, coltsfoot, marshmallow & horehound, drink as often as needed
Expectorant
Lung troubles
Phlegm, chest - syrup

Secondary Uses:
Appetite stimulant (especially with flu)
Diuretic
Gas
Perspiration - promotes
Purgative - gentle (large doses)
Stimulant - mild
Tonic
Wheezing - syrup
Worms - destroys & expels (powdered leaves)

Other Possible Uses:
Fever
Gas
Hay fever
Immune system - boosts
Placenta - helps expel
Sinusitis
Throat

External Uses:
Boils - dissolves
Coughs - lozenge
Hoarseness – lozenge

- Lozenge: 1-1/3 cup dried leaves steeped in 2 cups boiling water. Strain. Add 2 cups honey, 4 cups brown sugar and 1 tsp. cream of tartar. Heat to 220 degrees Fahrenheit. Add 1 tsp. butter and melt without stirring. Remove from heat, add 1 tsp. lemon juice and pour into hot buttered pans. Mark into squares and cool.
- Syrup: Use fresh green leaves and sugar.
- Stimulates the central nervous system.
- Stimulates the stomach to secrete digestive fluids and bile flow. Drink 30 minutes before meals for all gastrointestinal effects.
- May stop high and low blood sugar reactions after eating high carbohydrate meals and snacks.

Horseradish

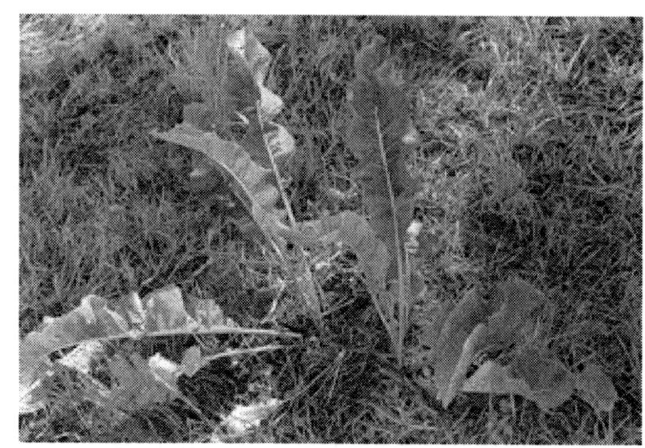

Cochlearia Amoracia
Mustard Family
Part Used: Root
Habitat: Britain; Europe.

Also known as: Great Raifort; Mountain Radish; Red Cole

Dosage: 5 - 20 grains

- Do not take in large quantities - may cause vomiting.
- May cause diarrhea and excessive sweating.

Primary Uses:
Antiseptic
Circulation
Coughs - with honey & warm water, especially after flu
Digestion, languid - with orange peel, nutmeg & wine
Diuretic
Dropsy
Expectorant
Scurvy
Stimulant
Whooping cough - with vinegar & glycerin
Worms - one of the best

Secondary Uses:
Asthma - with honey

Other Possible Uses:
Antibiotic
Arthritis
Gout
Kidneys
Lung infections
Rheumatism
Saliva - produces
Spleen
Stomachic
Tonic
Urinary infections

External Uses:
Rheumatism - poultice (overuse may cause blisters on skin)

Horsetail

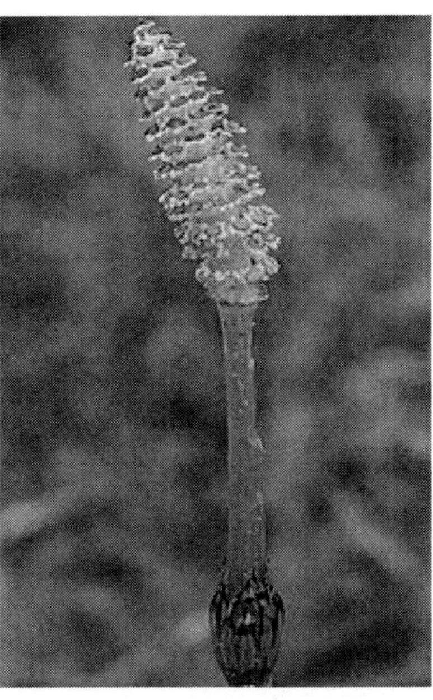

Equisetum arvense
Horsetail Family
Parts Used: Herb, Aerial parts of non-fruiting stems
Habitat: Britain; temperate northern regions.

Also known as: Bottle Brush; Dutch Rushes; Paddock Pipes; Pewterwort; Queue de Cheval; Scouring Rush; Shave Grass; Silica

Dosage: 60 grains

- May damage liver due to thiaminase poisoning.
- **Do not give to children under 2 years old.**
- Use caution with high blood pressure or cardiac disease.
- Extended use may cause kidney or heart damage.
- Contains nicotine.
- Avoid in presence of prostate cancer - may encourage growth of cancer cells.
- **Do not use during pregnancy - may cause birth defects from the high selenium content.**

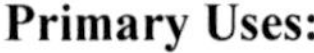

Primary Uses:
Astringent
Bladder problems
Bones - strengthen (broken ones too)
Connective tissue - heals & strengthens
Diuretic
Hair- strengthens & eliminates oil
Increases calcium absorption
Kidney problems - especially stones
Nails - strengthens
Skin - promotes healthy & eliminates oil
Teeth - strengthens

Secondary Uses:
Arthritis
Bedwetting & urinary incontinence
Dropsy
Gallbladder problems
Gravel
Hemorrhoids
Inflammation
Urinary ulcers

Other Possible Uses:
Bronchitis
Cooling
Emmenagogue - strong decoction
Heart - strengthen
Hemorrhaging
Lungs - strengthens
Muscle cramps
Osteoporosis
Prostate disorders
Rickets
Spitting blood
Stomach acidity - ashes of plant 3 -10 grains

External Uses:
Burns - poultice
Eyelids, swelling
Inflammation - juice
Wounds, bleeding - poultice

- Dried bunches of stems may be used for cleaning metal, especially pewter.
- May be eaten as a vegetable.
- Contains silica - strengthens connective tissue and combats arthritis.

Hyssop

Hyssopus officinalis
Mint Family
Parts Used: Leaves, Tops
Habitat: Mediterranean countries; North America; southern Europe.

Also known as: Isopo; Ysopo; Yssop

Dosage: 60 grains

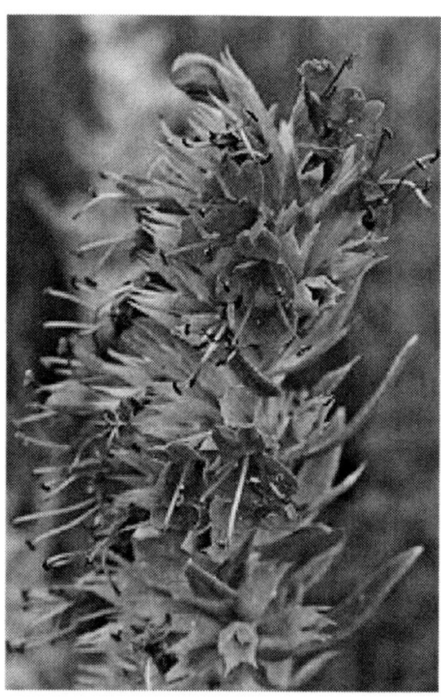

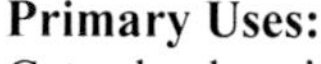

Primary Uses:
Catarrh, chronic
Chest complaints
Congestion
Expectorant

Secondary Uses:
Appetite stimulant
Asthma - green tops boiled in soup
Colds
Fever
Gas
Perspiration - produces
Sinuses
Stimulant

Other Possible Uses:
Anti-viral
Blood pressure - regulates
Circulation, problems
Epilepsy
Gout
Indigestion
Obesity
Rheumatism - tea from fresh green tops, several times a day

External Uses:
Aromatic
Bruises - leaves
Burns - wash
Cold sores
Cuts - green herb, bruised, heals quickly
Lice - oil
Rheumatism, muscular - leaves (also bath)
Skin irritation - wash
Throat, sore
Wounds

- Used to flavor liquors.

Juniper

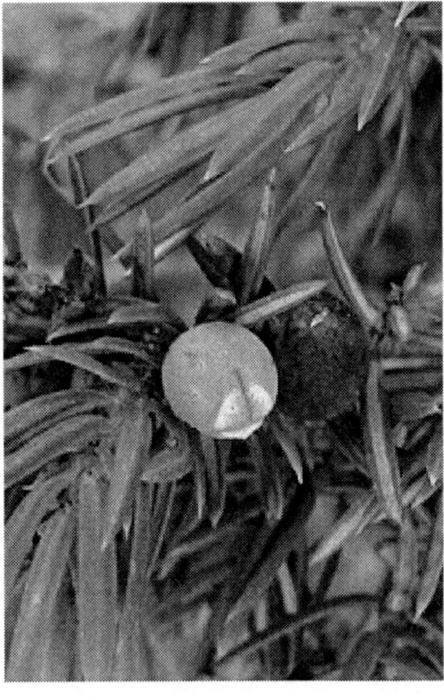

Juniperus communis
Conifer Family
Part Used: Berries, ripe and dried
Habitat: Europe; north Africa; North America; north Asia.

Also known as: Enebro; Gemeiner Wachholder; Geneva; Genevrier; Gin Plant; Ginberry; Ginepro; Horse Savin

Dosage: 60 grains

- Large doses may irritate bladder and urinary passages.
- May interfere with iron and other mineral absorption.
- **Do not use during pregnancy**.

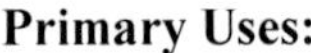

Primary Uses:
Bladder disease - oil
Diuretic - oil
Gas, with cramps - oil
Gout
Inflammation
Kidney disease - oil

Secondary Uses:
Cystitis
Digestive problems
Gallstones
Indigestion - oil
Rheumatism
Stomach - oil

Other Possible Uses:
Appetite stimulant - small doses
Asthma
Blood sugar levels - regulates
Cardiac dropsy - stimulating diuretic, spirits
Congestion
Depressant
Fever
Leucorrhoea
Obesity
Prostate disorders
Scrofula - berries (tuberculosis symptoms with swollen lymph glands)
Sedative

External Uses:
Flies on wounds, animals - oil mixed with lard
Stimulant, local - oil
Wounds, animals - oil mixed with lard

- Cooling Mixture: Mix 1 tsp. juniper decoction with 1 cup raspberry puree and freeze until slushy. Beat one egg white until stiff and fold into the mixture. Put into containers and freeze 2 hours. Serve with fresh mint. (To cool down in hot weather)
- Used to make gin.
- Boxes made of juniper are great for keeping out insects due to the oil in the wood.

Kava Kava

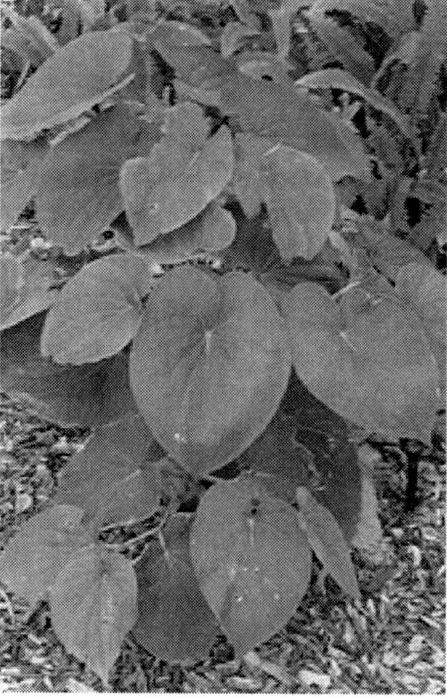

Piper Methysticum
Black Pepper Family
Part Used: Dried Root, peeled and divided
Habitat: Australia; Polynesia; Sandwich Islands; South Sea Islands.

Also known as: Ava; Ava Pepper; Ava Root; Awa Root; Intoxicating Pepper; Kava; Kave Pepper; Kawa Kawa

Dosage: 1 - 15 grains

- Long-term use may damage liver.
- Do not use more than 4 - 6 months consecutively.
- Do not use with alcohol or any medications that affects liver function, especially acetaminophen.
- Discontinue if notice signs of liver toxicity: fatigue, nausea, loss of appetite, pain in upper right abdomen, dark urine or yellowing of the eyes.
- Do not use in presence of hepatitis or cirrhosis
- Do not use with antidepressants, psychiatric medicines, sedatives or tranquilizers.
- **Do not use during pregnancy or while nursing.**
- Aggravates Parkinson's disease - causes twitches and weakness.
- Do not drive after taking.
- Avoid 2 weeks prior to surgery.

Primary Uses:
Anxiety
Bedwetting
Diuretic
Gonorrhea
Insomnia
Leucorrhoea
Nervousness
Restlessness
Sedative
Stress
Vaginitis

Secondary Uses:
Analgesic
Bronchitis
Cramps, muscular
Depression, anxiety related
Gout
Headache
Kidneys, pain
Narcotic - mild
Restless Leg Syndrome
Rheumatism
Sex drive, diminished
Urinary tract infections, pain

External Uses:
Analgesic
Anesthetic - local
Toothache

- Relieves urinary and kidney pain as urine is excreted from the body - lasts 24 hours.
- Non addictive.
- Promotes goodwill and relaxation.

Lady's Mantle

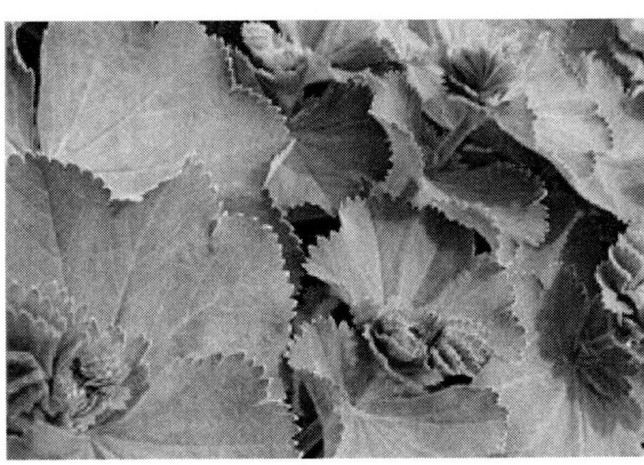

Alchemilla vulgaris
Rose Family
Parts Used: Herb, Root
Habitat: American Andes; Britain; Europe; North America; northern and western Asia; Scotch Highlands.

Also known as: Bear's Foot; Leontopodium; Lion's Foot; Nine Hooks; Stellaria

Dosage: 60 grains

- Contracts blood vessels.

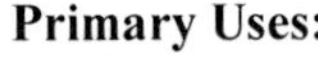

Primary Uses:
Astringent
Hemorrhaging - decoction
Menstruation, excessive - infusion
Vomiting blood
Wounds, internal - decoction (one of the best)

Secondary Uses:
Contracts tissues & blood vessels
Convulsive diseases - tincture of leaves
Purging, violent - halts

Other Possible Uses:
Appetite stimulant
Breasts, sagging - helps correct

External Uses:
Acne, chronic - infusion
Breasts, sagging - helps correct
Bruises
Douche - soothing
Gangrene - heals without leaving any behind
Inflammations
Sleep - placed under pillow
Wounds, deep - dries up
Wounds - heals by promoting cell growth (one of the best)

- Arabian women believe lady's mantle restores beauty and youth.

Lady's Slipper

Cypripedium pubescens
Orchid Family
Part Used: Root
Habitat: United States.

Also known as: American Valerian; Cypripedium Hirsutum; Nerve Root; Noah's Ark; Yellow Lady's Slipper

Dosage: 15 grains

- Large doses produce giddiness, restlessness, mental excitement and hallucinations.

Primary Uses:
Antispasmodic
Anxiety
D.T.'s, alcohol
Headaches, nervous
Hysteria
Insomnia
Irritability, nervous
Nerves
Pain
Spasms
Stimulant
Tension
Worms

Secondary Uses:
Cramps
Hypochondria
Psychedelic
Stimulant
Worms

- This herb is especially hard to find, as it is almost extinct due to wild crafting. If you find it, check the source to make sure it is grown for human consumption and not gathered in the wild.

Lavender

Lavendula officinalis
Mint Family
Part Used: Flowers
Habitat: Australia; England; France; Italy; western Mediterranean countries; Norway.

Also known as: Elfleaf; English Lavender; Nard; Nardus; Spike

Dosage: 10 - 30 grains

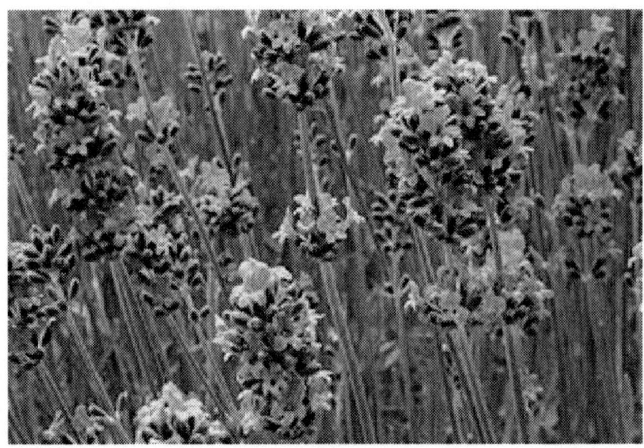

- **Do not overdose - too much is a narcotic poison and causes death by convulsions.**
- **Never take oil internally.**
- Best kept external. Use other herbs for the disorders where you can.
- Do not use in presence of gallstones or biliary tract obstruction - stimulates secretion of bile.
- **Do not use during pregnancy or while nursing.**
- Spanish lavender is stimulating - make certain you have the correct type of lavender.

Primary Uses:
Anxiety
Appetite stimulant
Depression
Epilepsy - with horehound, fennel, asparagus root and cinnamon
Faintness - oil
Headache
Heart, nervous palpitation
Insomnia
Nerves
Sedative
Stress
Tension

Secondary Uses:
Antiseptic
Antispasmodic
Convulsions
Gas
Memory loss
Muscle spasms
Vertigo

Other Possible Uses:
Catarrh
Colds
Coughs - steam
Liver
Mother's milk
Spleen
Stomach troubles - leaves
Strep throat - oil (gargle)
Vomiting - leaves

External Uses:
Acne
Antiseptic
Bronchitis - inhale oil vapors
Bruises
Burns - oil, prevents from infection, relieves pain & heals
Cuts - antibacterial
Douche
Eczema
Fatigue - bath
Fungus
Hair, greasy
Hoarseness - gargle
Lice
Pain - hot in bags applied locally
Psoriasis
Rheumatism
Sleep - bag under pillow
Sprains
Stings
Sunburn – 2x per day cool compresses, soaked in tea
Toothache
Wounds

- Lavender honey: Pour warm honey over 2 spikes of lavender. Cover and infuse for 2 weeks.
- Tea: 1 - 2 tsp. dried flowers to 1 cup hot (not boiling) water. Steep 5 - 10 minutes and strain.
- Sugar cube: 1 cube with 4 drops essential oil (maximum!).

Licorice

Glycyrrhiza glabra
Legume Family
Part Used: Root, dug in autumn once plant is 3 - 4 years old
Habitat: Southeast Europe; southwest Asia to Persia.

Also known as: Licorish; Liquorice; Lycorys; Sweet Root

Dosage: 10 - 30 grains

- **Do not use during pregnancy.**
- Do not use in presence of diabetes, glaucoma, heart disease, high blood pressure, severe menstrual problems, or history of stroke.
- Do not use more than 7 days in a row or may result in high blood pressure even in people with previously normal blood pressure.
- Large doses leech potassium from the body.
- Large doses may cause temporary loss of vision.
- May cause water retention and bloating.
- Do not take with lithium - causes serious mineral imbalances.
- Do not use with diuretics - causes dangerous potassium loss and kidney damage, especially with calcium carbonate.
- Do not use licorice candy - not the same as licorice root. It will not work.
- Neutralizes high blood pressure medication.
- Do not use with steroids - increases both medicinal and undesirable side effects.
- Raises blood pressure and may result in heart irregularities.
- Do not use in presence of liver disease, diabetes, glaucoma or kidney disease.
- May cause fluid retention, high blood pressure and loss of potassium.
- Do not use in presence of estrogen sensitive disorders - promotes conversion of testosterone to estrogen.
- Avoid in presence of erectile dysfunction or male infertility.

Primary Uses:
Anti-inflammatory
Bronchitis
Chest complaints
Coughs
Expectorant
Heartburn
Hoarseness - with rosewater
Indigestion
Inflammation, internal & tissue - soothes
Laryngitis
Phlegm - increases fluidity
Respiratory problems
Throat, sore
Ulcers, peptic

Secondary Uses:
Adrenal gland function - promotes
AIDS - may stop & heal
Allergies
Antiviral
Asthma
Cancer, breast, prostate - protects against arsenic compounds, nicotine & caffeine
Celiac disease
Colitis, ulcerative
Colon - cleanses
Crohn's disease
Fatigue, chronic - take 1 month minimum
Fever, children
Fibromyalgia
Hepatitis - protects liver & promotes healing, keeps from spreading
HIV - may stop & heal
Hypoglycemia
Irritable Bowel Syndrome
Laxative - mild
Lupus
Lyme Disease - prevents progression & counteracts fatigue
Premenstrual Syndrome
Spasms, muscular - decreases

Thirst - prevents, excellent
Tonic
Licorice
continued

Other Possible Uses:
Arthritis, pain
Bladder ailments
Depression
Detox
Emphysema
Herpes virus
Kidney ailments
Nutritive
Rejuvenative

External Uses:
Canker sores
Diaper rash
Eczema - cream
Itching
Shingles - cream
Skin, burning

- Syrup: 1 tsp. linseed, 1 ounce licorice root and ¼ pound raisins. Put in 2 quarts water and simmer down to 1 quart. Add ¼ pound brown sugar or brown sugar candy and 1 tbls. white vinegar or lemon juice.
- Used in stout beers for color and thickness.
- Used by singers to strengthen their throats.
- Diabetics may safely take sugar of licorice.
- Used to disguise the taste of bitter medicines.

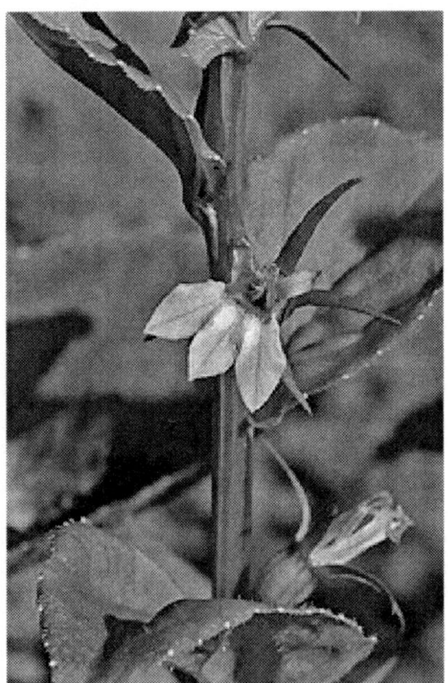

Lobelia

Lobelia inflata
Lobelia Family
Parts Used: Dried Flowering Herb, Seeds
Habitat: Canada; Kamchatka; northern United States; dry areas.

Also known as: Asthma Weed; Bladderpod; Eyebright; Gagroot; Indian Tobacco; Pukeweed; Vomitwort

Dosage: 1 - 5 grains

- Do not use as an emetic.
- **Poisonous in large doses even when absorbed through the epidermis.**
- Overdose causes suppressed breathing, coma, narcotic poisoning, nausea, cold sweats and depression.
- Do not misuse.

Primary Uses:
Antispasmodic
Asthma
Bronchitis
Colic
Convulsions
Coughs
Diphtheria
Epilepsy
Expectorant
Fever
Laryngitis
Perspiration - produces
Relaxant
Tetanus
Throat, sore

Other Possible Uses:
Abscesses
Hysteria
Mucus
Pain
Phlegm
Sleep
Syphilis
Worms

External Uses:
Bites
Inflammation - poultice
Poison ivy
Ulcers - poultice

This can be a dangerous herb, as it is poisonous and the poison can enter through unbroken skin. Be careful when handling and watch the dosage.

Ma Huang

Ephedra vulgaris
Gnetum Family
Part Used: Top of plant
Habitat: Japan; southern Siberia; west central China.

Also known as: Ephedra; Ephedrine; Epitonin; Mormon Tea

Dosage: ½ - 1 grain

- Do not use if you have a history of panic attacks.
- Do not use in presence of glaucoma, heart disease, high blood pressure, enlarged prostate, diabetes, lupus, hardening arteries, anxiety, nervous disorders or if taking an monoamine oxidase inhibitor.
- Will cause increased heart rate, pain in the chest, panic and racing pulse when taken with caffeine or other herbal stimulants. Many have been hospitalized or even killed from the combination of this herb with one cup of coffee alone.
- **Do not use during pregnancy or while nursing**. May trigger early labor.
- Do not give to young children or anyone with liver, heart or kidney disease.
- May cause kidney stones.
- Raises blood sugar levels.
- Tolerance will develop.
- Dangerously elevates blood pressure.
- Check labels - disguised as Epitonin, jointfir, sea grape, desert tea, popotillo, herbal ecstasy, teamaster's tea, yellow astringent and yellow horse.
- May cause ephedra overdose in combination with cold remedies.
- Interacts with high blood pressure and heart disease medications, diuretics and monoamine oxidase inhibitors.
- May cause high blood pressure, stroke, seizures and sudden death.
- Increases heart rate.

Primary Uses:
Allergies
Asthma
Bronchial spasms - dilates bronchial tubes
Colds
Expectorant
Nerve stimulant resembling adrenaline
Respiratory complaints

Secondary Uses:
Appetite suppressant
Decongestant
Hay fever
Influenza, low blood pressure
Mucous membrane swelling
Pneumonia, low blood pressure

Other Possible Uses:
Antispasmodic
Diuretic
Rheumatism

- Use of the whole herb reduces the risks and side effects, but does not eliminate them. The individual constituents when taken alone cause the majority of the problems.

Marshmallow

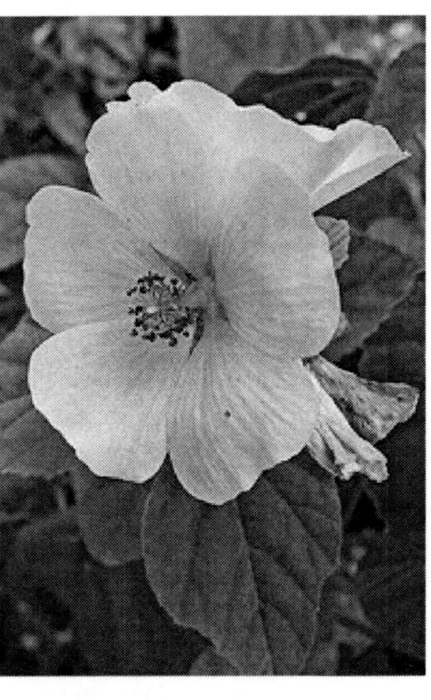

Althaea officinalis
Mallow Family
Parts Used: Leaves, Root, Flowers
Habitat: England; Europe; Scotland; in salt marshes, damp meadows, ditches, by the sea and on banks of tidal rivers.

Also known as: Althaea Root; Cheeses; Mallards; Mauls; Mortification Root; Schloss Tea

Dosage: 30 - 60 grains; 1 tbls. to 8 ounces hot water

Primary Uses:
Asthma
Bladder infection, pain & disorders
Bronchitis - boiled in wine or milk
Colds
Colitis (one of the best)
Coughs - boiled in wine or milk
Expectorant
Gastrointestinal disorders
Indigestion
Laryngitis
Lungs - boiled in wine or milk
Mucous membranes, inflamed
Sinuses
Sore throat
Stomach inflammation
Ulcers, peptic
Urine pain
Whooping cough - boiled in wine or milk

Secondary Uses:
Crohn's disease
Diuretic
Intestines
Kidney disorders
Stomach pain

Other Possible Uses:
Genitals
Gums
Melancholia
Mouth
Teeth
Throat

External Uses:
Bruises
Douche
Eczema
Eyewash
Genitals
Hair, dry
Inflammation - warm poultice
Mastitis
Pain
Psoriasis
Rectal - sitz bath
Skin - bath
Sprains
Staph sores
Wound discharge

- Expels excesses fluids and mucous from the body.
- Forms a protective layer on the stomach lining completely and lowers acid levels.

Milk Thistle

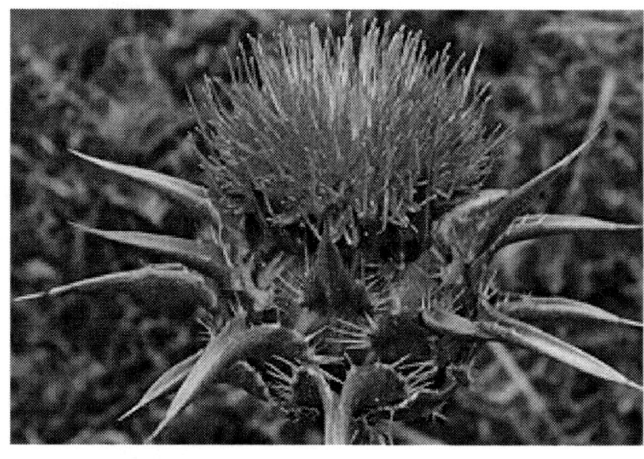

Silybum Marianum
Composite Family
Parts Used: Whole herb, Root, Leaves, Seeds (dried), Hulls
Habitat: Australia; California; Europe; Mediterranean countries.

Also known as: Marian Thistle; Mary Thistle; Silymarin; Wild Artichoke

Dosage: No standard dosage

- May decrease effectiveness of Indinavir (for HIV and AIDS).
- May reduce effectiveness of oral contraceptives.

Primary Uses:
Alcoholism, liver problems
Bile - increases production of
Cirrhosis - take 8 weeks minimum
Hepatitis - take 8 weeks minimum
Jaundice - infusion - take 8 weeks minimum
Liver - protects, heals, stimulates production of new cells - take 8 weeks minimum
Liver obstructions - removes - infusion

Secondary Uses:
Acne
Cancer
Constipation
Crohn's disease
Diabetes, insulin resistant - helps use insulin
High cholesterol
Irritable Bowel Syndrome
Parkinson's disease - slows
Psoriasis - lessens frequency
Spleen obstructions - removes - infusion
Stones - breaks & expels - infusion

Other Possible Uses:
Adrenal disorders
Antioxidant
Detox
Gallbladder disease & stones
Immune system, weakened
Inflammation, internal - soothes
Kidneys - protects

External Uses:
Cancer - decoction
Psoriasis

- The purple flowering heads may be eaten fresh or as a vegetable, similar to an artichoke.
- Increases the production of bile, which also removes the byproducts that cause cancer.
- Prevents damage to liver cells and helps liver regenerate from hepatitis, cirrhosis, mushroom poisoning, etc.
- May be taken during pregnancy or while nursing. (Seek medical advice first).

Mistletoe

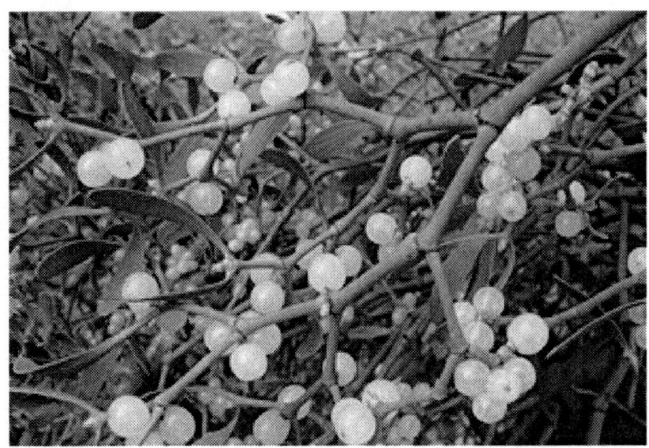

Viscum album
Mistletoe Family
Parts Used: Leaves, Young twigs
Habitat: Worldwide, on branches of trees.

Also known as: Allheal; Birdlime; Birdlime Mistletoe; Devil's Fuge; European Mistletoe; Golden Bough; Herbe de la Croix; Holywood; Lignum Crucis; Loranthus; Mulberry Mistletoe; Mystyldene; Thunderbesem; Witches Broom; Wood of the Cross

Dosage: 15 - 30 grains

- Do not use the berries.
- Do not take with a monoamine oxidase inhibitor.
- Do not use with heart medications - may cause cardiac depression.
- Do not use with high blood pressure medications - may cause dangerous drop in blood pressure.
- Do not take with sedatives.
- **Do not use during pregnancy or while nursing.**

Primary Uses:
Antispasmodic
Delirium
Epilepsy
Heart disease
Hemorrhaging, internal
High blood pressure
Hysteria
Nerves
Sedative
Tonic
Tranquilizer
Urinary disorders

Secondary Uses:
Cancer*
Convulsions
Menstrual pain & spasms
Menstruation, excessive

Other Possible Uses:
Arthritis
Headaches
Heart rate - slows
Migraines
Paralysis

* Used as an injection in Europe. It poisons cancer cells and stimulates the immune system, allowing tumors to become sensitive to the immune system. Increases NK and T-cells, and increases the production of beneficial free radicals.

- The berries have been reported to have caused the deaths of two children. These are the only cases of poison documented at this time of writing. The berries are reported to cause nausea, vomiting, abnormally high or low blood pressure, seizures, slow heart beat and the possibility of death.
- Use Mulberry Mistletoe, which has feathery leaves, yellow flowers in clusters of 3 and round, sticky, white berries. American mistletoe has white flowers and rounded leaves and is the kind used in Christmas decorations - this is the toxic one.

Mullein

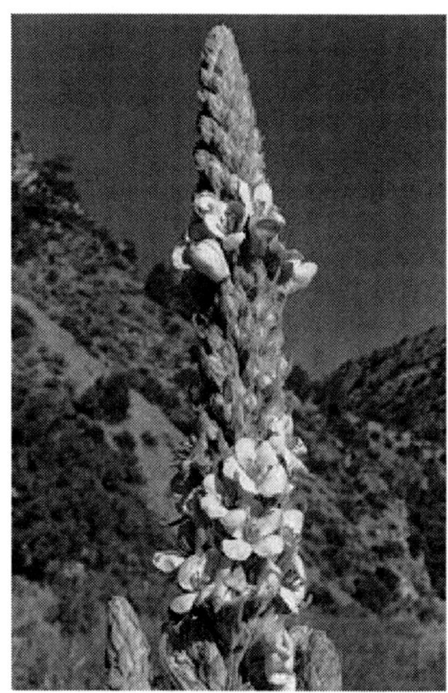

Verbascum thapsus
Spinach Family (some sources claim Figwort Family)
Parts Used: Leaves, Flowers, Root
Habitat: Britain, on hedge-banks, roadsides and waste areas; Europe, North America, especially eastern United States; temperate Asia.

Also known as: Aaron's Rod; Beggar's Blanket; Blanket Herb; Bullock's Lungwort; Candlewick; Clot; Clown's Lungwort; Cuddy's Lungs; Doffle; Duffle; Feltwort; Flannel Plant; Fluffweed; Hag's Taper; Graveyard Dust; Hare's Beard; Jacob's Staff; Jupiter's Staff; Lady's Foxglove; Mullein Dock; Old Man's Flannel; Orange Mullein; Our Lady's Flannel; Peter's Staff; Rag Paper; Range-Flowered Mullein; Shepherd's Clubs; Shepherd's Herb; Shepherd's Staff; Torches; Velvetback; Velvet Dock; Velvet Plant; White Mullein; Wild Ice Leaf; Woollen

Dosage: 30 - 60 grains; 1 tbls. to 8 ounce hot water

- **Do not use during pregnancy or while nursing.**
- The seeds are toxic and cause poisoning.
- Contains tannins.

Primary Uses:
Asthma - smoke
Astringent
Bowels, bleeding - with milk
Breathing, difficulty
Bronchitis
Chest problems, all
Constipation
Coughs, hacking - smoke or boiled in milk
Diarrhea - with milk
Expectorant - infusion with milk
Glandular swelling
Hay fever
Hemorrhaging
Hemorrhoids
Inflammation, internal (all)
Insomnia
Laxative
Lungs, bleeding
Migraine - tincture with wine (8-10 drops) frequently (water may be substituted)
Pain
Sedative
Sleep

Secondary Uses:
Diuretic
Flu
Gastrointestinal disorders
Hoarseness
Inflammation, throat
Sinuses

Other Possible Uses:
Antispasmodic
Dysentery
Stomach cramps
Whooping cough

External Uses:
Burns - distilled water
Cuts
Earache - oil (2-3 drops, 3x per day)
Hemorrhoids - poultice
Lung irritation - smoke
Skin - softens
Warts
Wounds

- Restricts tissue and reduces bleeding externally. Also helps internally to prevent diarrhea.

Myrrh

Commiphora myrrha
Frankincense Family
Part Used: Resin
Habitat: Arabia; Somaliland.

Also known as: Balsamodendron Myrrha; Bowl; Commiphora Myrrha; Didin; Didthin; Gun Myrrh Tree; Karan; Mirra; Morr; Mukkul

Dosage: 10 - 30 grains

- **Do not use during pregnancy.**
- Do not overdose.
- Avoid in presence of heavy periods - increases menstrual flow.
- Large amounts may produce violent laxative effects and cause vomiting and accelerated heart beat.

Primary Uses:
Appetite stimulant
Astringent
Colds
Coughs
Emmenagogue - direct (one of the best)
Expectorant
Flu, stomach (excellent)
Stimulant
Stomachic
Tonic
Ulcers - with goldenseal (half & half)

Secondary Uses:
Bronchitis
Poisons - helps absorb (charcoal capsule are even better, or a combination)
White blood cell count - increases
Worms

Other Possible Uses:
Gas
Mother's Milk

External Uses:
Analgesic
Anti-inflammatory, mouth & throat
Antiseptic
Astringent
Bacteria in mouth - gargle
Bad breath
Bedsores
Canker sores
Cuts
Deodorizer
Disinfectant
Douche
Embalming
Eye infections
Gingivitis
Gums, spongy & soft
Hemorrhoids
Mouth sores - wash
Pain
Periodontal disease
Sores - balm
Strep throat
Swelling
Teeth
Tooth decay
Thrush
Ulcers - tincture
Wounds

- Does not coat throat and mouth - only reduces inflammation and soreness in throat and mouth problems.
- Dilute the tincture to prevent burning sensations.

Nettles

Urtica Dioica
Nettle Family
Parts Used: Leaves, Root
Habitat: Andes; Australia; southern Africa; temperate regions in the northern hemisphere.

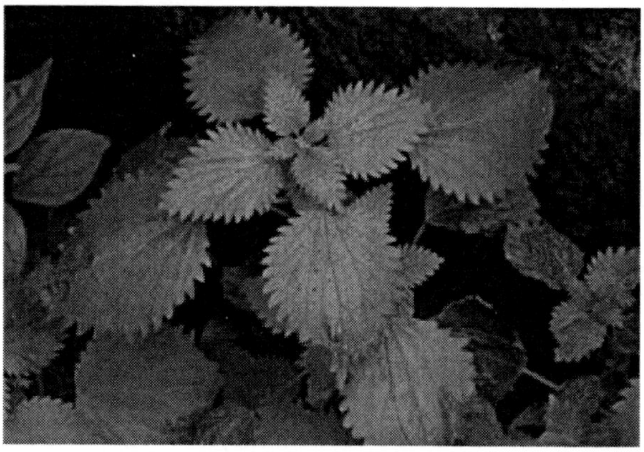

Also known as: Stinging Nettles

Dosage: 30 - 60 grains

- Do not eat uncooked plant.
  May damage kidneys and cause symptoms of poisoning.
- May remove potassium from body.
- Causes skin irritation before dried.
- **Do not use during pregnancy or while nursing.**
- Do not use in presence of fluid retention from conjunctive heart failure or kidney disease.
- Do not use if coming down with the flu or if already have the flu.
- May interact with medications for diabetes, high blood pressure, sedatives and inflammations - use caution. There are no reports to date though.

Primary Uses:
Allergies, hay fever - increases production of T-cells (food allergies too)
Anemia - contains iron, vitamin C & chlorophyll
Anti-inflammatory - leaf
Arthritis
Astringent
Asthma
Bowel disorders
Colon disorders
Cystitis
Diarrhea
Diuretic
Eczema
Expectorant
Hemorrhoids - tea
Lupus
Pain
Poisoning from hemlock, henbane & belladonna - nettle seeds
Urinary disorders
Uterine - tonic
Venomous bites - seeds
Worms
BPH (Benign Prostatic Hypertrophy) - decreases rate of cell division in prostate & eases urine flow
Diabetes - prevents with fasting
Gout
Hay fever
High blood sugar
Obesity - with fasting (seeds)
Prostate problems - root only
Sex drive, diminished, men & women

Other Possible Uses:
Complexion
Detox
Migraine
Mother's milk - increases

External Uses:
Balding - hair tonic (also lotion every night)
Hair, greasy
Hives - especially from shellfish (by its caffeic malic acid)
Raise skin blisters - fresh leaves
Shampoo - healthy hair
Sores
Yeast infections

Secondary Uses:

- Fed to poultry to harden eggshells.

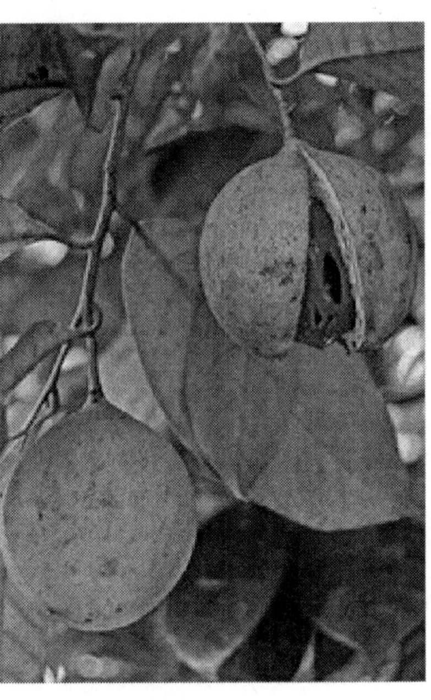

Nutmeg

Myristica fragrans
Nutmeg Family
Parts Used: Dried Kernel of Seed
Habitat: Banda Islands; French Guiana; Malayan Archipelago; Molucca Islands; Sumatra.

Also known as: Myristica; Myristica Aromata; Myristica Officinalis; Nux Moschata

Dosage: 5 - 20 grains

- **Do not use excessive amounts - will make you VERY sick - unbearable and unbelievable pain and nausea.**

Primary Uses:
Digestion - promotes

Secondary Uses:
Gas
Nausea
Vomiting

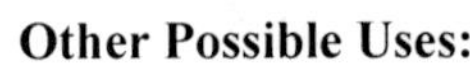
Other Possible Uses:
Narcotic
Saliva – produces

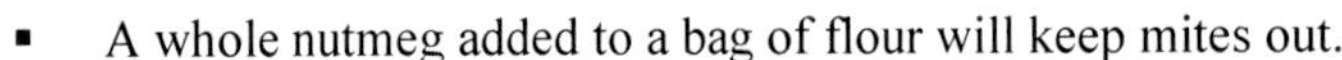

- A whole nutmeg added to a bag of flour will keep mites out.

Oregon Grape

Berberis aquifolium
Barberry Family
Parts Used: Root bark, Leaves
Habitat: Western United States.

Also known as: Alegrita; Berberry; California Barberry; Holly Leaved Barberry; Japonica; Mountain Grape; Mountain Holly; Pepperidge; Rocky Mountain Grape; Sourberry; Sowberry; Trailing Grape; Wild Oregon Grape; Yellow Root

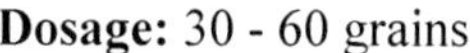

Dosage: 30 - 60 grains

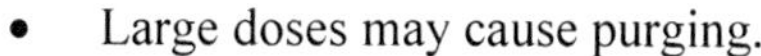

- Large doses may cause purging.
- Use caution with anti-anxiety medications - mildly sedative.
- May lower blood sugar.
- May irritate stomach and aggravate chronic heartburn.
- **May cause uterine contractions - Do not use during pregnancy**.
- Do not use more than 3 weeks consecutively.

Primary Uses:
Acne
Detox, blood & liver
Digestion - improves
Jaundice
Liver, sluggish - cleanses
Psoriasis
Skin problems - by cleansing liver
Tonic

Secondary Uses:
Bowels, sluggish
Constipation - with cascara sagrada
Diarrhea, bacterial dysentery
Gallbladder - stimulates
Gastritis
Mucus, chronic complaints
Syphilis

Other Possible Uses:
Boils
E. coli - inhibits ability to attach to human cells
Indigestion
Rheumatism
Scrofula (tuberculosis), early stages
Typhoid, early stages

External Uses:
Acne
Astringent - root
Eczema
Local anesthetic - root
Psoriasis
Rashes, allergic
Skin – heals

- Extracts and compresses are applied 3 times per day.
- All species are used interchangeably.

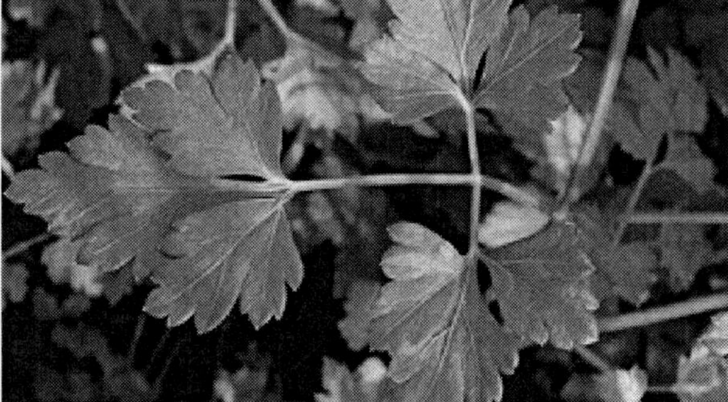

Parsley

Carum petroselinum
Carrot Family
Parts Used: Roots, Seeds
Habitat: Eastern Mediterranean; England; Scotland.

Also known as: Devil's Oatmeal; Percely; Persele; Persely; Persil; Petersilie; Petroselinium; Rock Parsley

Dosage: 60 grains

- Large doses produce low blood pressure, deafness, giddiness and paralysis.
- **May be fatal to parrots and some small birds.**

Primary Uses:
Bad breath
Bedwetting
Bladder function
Digestion - stimulates
Diuretic
Dropsy
Gas
Goiter
Halitosis
Indigestion
Jaundice
Kidney - function & stones, tea (one of the best)
Liver function
Lung function
Menstrual disorders
Obesity
Rheumatism
Stomach, pain
Thyroid function
Tumors - prevents cell multiplication
Worms

Secondary Uses:
Alcoholism
Aphrodisiac
Appetite - stimulates
Bodybuilding
Brain, function
Colic
Coughs
Fever
Gallstones
Gonorrhea
Gout
High blood pressure
Intestines
Mother's milk
Nerves
Prostate disorders
Spleen

External Uses:
Insect stings - poultice
Skin, itchy
Swelling - poultice

Passion Flower

Passiflora incarnate
Passion Flower Family
Part Used: Dried Herb, collected after some berries have matured
Habitat: Southeastern United States.

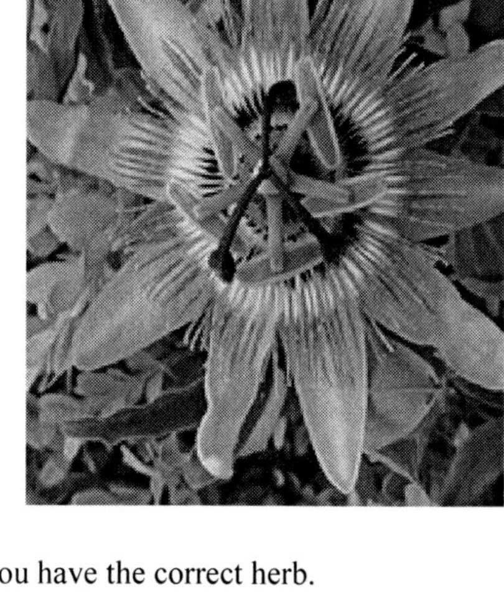

Also known as: Apricot Vine; Blue Passion Flower; Granadilla; Maracoc; Maypops; Passion Vine

Dosage: 3 - 10 grains

- Increases the effect of alcohol and psychoactive drugs such as sedatives and tranquilizers.
- Causes drowsiness.
- Depresses the central nervous system.
- Do not use with monoamine oxidase inhibitors.
- **Do not use during pregnancy - stimulates uterine muscles.**
- Passiflora caerulea contains cyanide - make sure you have the correct herb.
- Do not give to children under 2 and give in lower doses to children 2 - 12 and adults over 65.

Primary Uses:
Anxiety
Emotional upset, extreme
Hyperactivity
Hysteria
Insomnia, nervous
Nerves, pain
Restless Leg Syndrome
Restlessness
Sedative
Stress

Secondary Uses:
Attention Deficit Disorder
Diarrhea
Diuretic
Epilepsy
Headache, nervous
High blood pressure
Kidney complaints
Narcotic
Sex drive, diminished - men & women
Shingles

- Increases testosterone.
- Useful in stopping the chemical reactions that cause nausea and vomiting due to withdrawal from cocaine, heroin or opiates.
- Increases effectiveness of some sleep aids.
- May be used as a sedative by people addicted to drugs and alcohol.

Pau D'Arco

Tabebuia impetiginosa
Trumpet Creeper Family
Part Used: Dried inner bark
Habitat: South America.

Also known as: Lapacho

Dosage: 300 mg, 3x a day

- Do not use with anticoagulants - causes excessive bleeding and intensifies effect.
- High doses cause nausea, vomiting and excessive, uncontrolled bleeding.
- Only use for one week at a time to avoid health risks.
- **Do not use during pregnancy or while nursing.**
- May interfere with cancer medications.
- Always use the whole herb.

Primary Uses:
Antibacterial
Anti fungal
Cancer - anti tumor properties
Candida (yeast infection)
Detox
Digestion
Fungal infections
High blood sugar
Leukemia
Parasitic infection, Espchagas' disease (common in Texas)
River blindness (Schistosomiasis, parasitic infection)
Tumors
Ulcers, gastric & peptic

Secondary Uses:
AIDS
Allergies
Anti-inflammatory
Colds
Coughs, smokers
Diabetes - prevents glucose in urine
Lupus
Pain
Rheumatism

External Uses:
Athlete's foot
Boils
Fungal infections
Ringworm
Warts
Wounds
Yeast infection

- Increases effectiveness of chemotherapy while decreasing negative side effects.
- Helps against drug-resistant strains of malaria and Plasmodium falciparum.

Pennyroyal

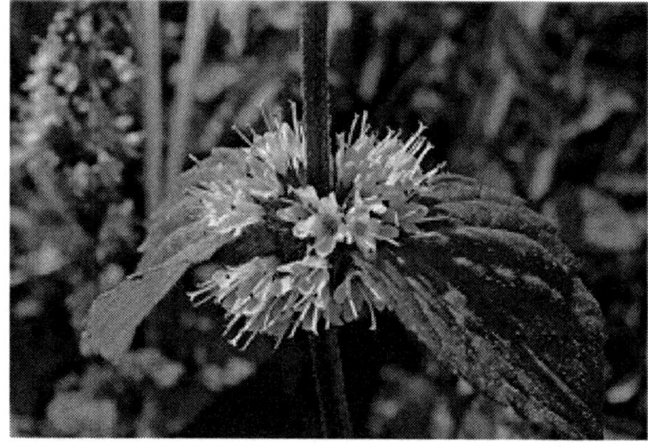

Mentha Pulegium
Mint Family
Part Used: Herb
Habitat: Asia; Europe.

Also known as: Lurk-in-the-ditch; Mosquito Plant; Orgam Tea; Organ Broth; Organs; Piliolerial; Pudding Grass; Pulegium; Run-by-the-ground; Squaw Mint; Tickweed

Dosage: 60 grains

- Do not use for more than one week at a time.
- **Do not use during pregnancy.**
- Large doses may produce nausea, vomiting and toxicity - may be fatal.
- Abortive - has resulted in hemorrhaging and serious complications for the mother.

Primary Uses:
Bronchitis
Colds - warm infusion
Coughs
Cramps, menstrual (due to suppressed menstruation)
Emmenagogue
Gas, pain
Griping
Labor - facilitates
Lungs - cleanses & clears, with honey
Menstrual problems - tea
Perspiration - produces, warm infusion
Phlegm - clears, with honey
Premenstrual Syndrome, especially bloating
Whooping cough - 1 spoon juice with sugar

Secondary Uses:
Detox
Diuretic
Giddiness
Gout
Headaches
Hysteria - water
Nervous problems - water
Stimulant
Stomach - warming (problems with fermentation)
Vertigo

Other Possible Uses:
Colic
Diarrhea
Jaundice
Nausea
Rheumatism
Sea sickness - leaves steeped in vinegar with a bit of wormwood & chamomile
Spasms

External Uses:
Aromatic
Bruises - green herb bruised (especially on eyes)
Faintness - applied to nostrils with vinegar
Fleas - prevents
Flies - prevents
Gnats - prevents
Insects - repellent for pets & people - a few drops oil on the animal or person
Mosquitoes - prevents
Moths - repels
Skin, itchy
Ticks – prevents

- Infusion: 1 ounce to 1 pint boiling water.
- Was once cast into water to purify it.
- Makes a great shampoo for humans and animals.
- The oil may be combined with equal parts of garlic oil and sprayed in hen houses and runs to keep ticks away. This mixture also works to rid dogs and cats of fleas when used as a bath. (Do not rinse off).

Peppermint

Mentha piperita
Mint Family
Part Used: Leaves
Habitat: America; England, in moist areas and wastelands; Europe.

Also known as: American Mint; Balm Mint; Brandy Mint; Curled Mint; Lammint; White Mint

Dosage: 60 grains

- May interfere with iron absorption.
- Do not use with Felodipine for high blood pressure or with Simuastatin for cholesterol.
- More than 2 drops of oil on the tongue may cause heartburn and digestive upset, even leading to seizures.
- Pure menthol is fatal in doses as small as 2 grams. Do not ever ingest! Even 1 tsp. can kill. Keep in mind - this is a major ingredient in peppermint oil.
- Do not put oil on chest or nose of any child under 5 years old - may cause choking.
- Oil will intensify symptoms of hiatal hernia.
- Oil stimulates release of bile.
- **Do not use the oil during pregnancy – causes relaxed uterus.**
- Do not use for morning sickness if you have any history of miscarriage.
- Do not use in presence of chronic heartburn.
- Do not use in presence of gallstone disorders.

Primary Uses:
Antispasmodic
Appetite - increases
Colds, slight - tea
Colic
Coughs, nagging
Cramps, abdominal
Diarrhea
Digestion - enhances by increasing stomach acidity
Dysentery
Gas, pain - spirit in hot water
Heart trouble & palpitation
Indigestion
Motion sickness - tea
Nausea - oil
Pain, abdominal - boiled in milk & drunk hot
Stomachic
Vomiting - oil

Secondary Uses:
Allergies, food
Burping - promotes
Chills
Colic
Crohn's disease
Dizziness
Fever
Food poisoning - oil, kills microorganisms
Gall stones - relieves spasms of bile duct
Headache - tea
Irritable Bowel Syndrome - blocks contractions
Muscle relaxer
Nervous disorders - infusion
Stimulant
Ulcers, peptic

Other Possible Uses:
Antibacterial
Cholera
Heartburn
Hysteria - infusion
Indigestion
Insomnia
Liver disorders
Migraine
Perspiration - induces
Raises internal heat

Rheumatism

External Uses:
Anesthetic, local - oil
Antiseptic - oil
Ants - repels
Aphids - repels
Bad
Headache - oil on forehead
Pain, spasms & strains
Stress - oil, applied to temples to relieve tension
Toothache & cavities - oil, mouthwash

- The oil is usually put on sugar cubes and herb is regularly mixed with other herbs for flavor.
- Rats hate peppermint oil - use soaked rags to plug holes.
- Stops the growth of salmonella bacteria and slows listeria.
- Used with purgatives to prevent griping.

Pleurisy

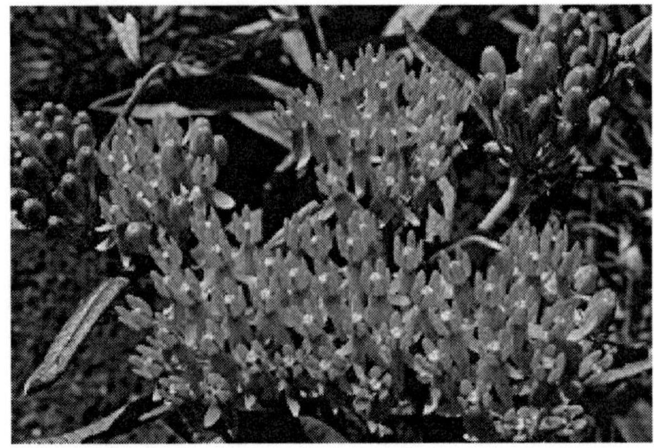

Asclepias tuberosa
Milkweed Family
Part Used: Root
Habitat: Africa; Canada; North America; South America.

Also known as: Butterfly Weed; Colic Root; Orange Milkweed; Pipple Root; Swallow Wort; Tuber Root; Wind Root

Dosage: 20 - 30 grains

- Large doses are emetic and have purgative effects.
- The fresh root may be dangerous.

Primary Uses:
Bronchitis
Chest complaints, all
Coughs, spasmodic
Expectorant - warm infusion, every hour
Gas
Inflammation, lungs
Pleurisy, difficulty breathing & pain (with angelica & sassafras)
Pneumonia
Throat, catarrh

Secondary Uses:
Antispasmodic
Diarrhea
Fever - with angelica & sassafras
Indigestion (rarely used)
Perspiration, produces - warm infusion every hour

Other Possible Uses:
Circulation - equalizes (with angelica & sassafras)
Diuretic
Dysentery
Eczema
Laxative
Rheumatism, acute & chronic
Tonic

- Infusion: 1 tsp. powder to 1 cup boiling water.

Poke

Phytolacca decandra
Pokeweed Family
Part Used: Root, dried
Habitat: Mediterranean; North America.

Also known as: American Nightshade; American Spinach; Branching Grape; Branching Phytolacca; Cancer-Root; Chongras; Coakum; Cocan; Crowberry; Inkberry; Jalap; Phytolacca Berry; Phytolacca Root; Phytolaccae Bacca; Phytolaccae Radix; Pigeon Berry; Pocan; Poke Berry; Poke Weed; Polkroot; Pokeroot; Red Ink Plant; Skoke; Virginian Poke

Dosage: 1 - 5 grains

- Do not use as emetic or risk death.
- **Do not eat raw leaves - POISON.** (Only the top-most leaves and young shoots are edible, and only during certain seasons - be very careful!)
- Overdoses cause considerable vomiting and purging, prostration, convulsions and death.

Primary Uses:
Bowels - regulates
Rheumatism, chronic - infused in spirits

Secondary Uses:
Emetic - slow with narcotic properties (10 grains)
Headache
Purgative - slow with narcotic properties (10 grains)
Tapeworm

Other Possible Uses:
Astringent
Cancer, breast
Detox
Dysentery
Leucorrhoea - tincture
Liver - regulates

External Uses:
Cancer - bath
Hemorrhoids - extract
Leucorrhoea - lotion
Psoriasis
Rheumatism - extract
Ringworm
Scabies
Skin diseases - ointment (may burn slightly)

- The purple stain from the berries cannot be "fixed", so it is not a good dye.
- Root decoction has been used in drenching cattle.
- If poultry eats too many of the berries, their flesh also becomes purgative to humans.

Primrose, Evening

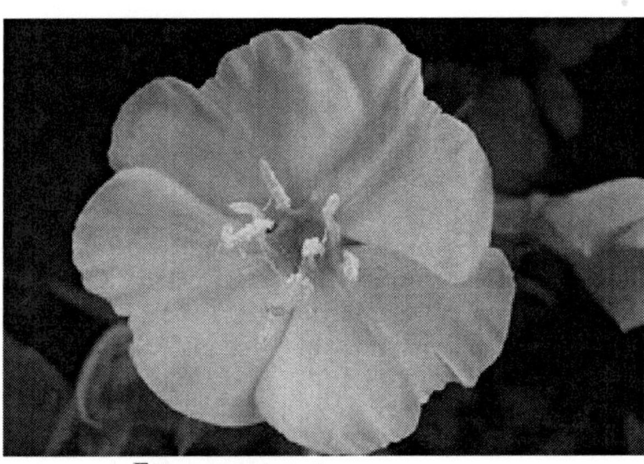

Oenothera biennis
Primrose Family
Parts Used: Bark, Leaves
Habitat: England; Europe; North America.

Also known as: Evening Primrose; Tree Primrose

Dosage: 5 - 30 grains

Primary Uses:
Acne
Bloating
Breast tenderness
Cramps
Eczema, especially infantile (cradle cap)
High blood pressure
Hot flashes
Irritability
Menopause
Menstrual bleeding - heavy
Premenstrual Syndrome
Skin disorders & health

Secondary Uses:
Alcoholism
Arthritis
Asthma
Astringent
Estrogen promoter
High cholesterol
Liver, torpid
Sedative

Other Possible Uses:
Anxiety
Gastro-intestinal disorders
Hyperactivity
Indigestion
Multiple sclerosis
Nervine
Pain
Schizophrenia - helps
Whooping cough

External Uses:
Face wash

- Not to be mistaken with the Primrose *Primula vulgaris*, which has emetic properties.

Psyllium

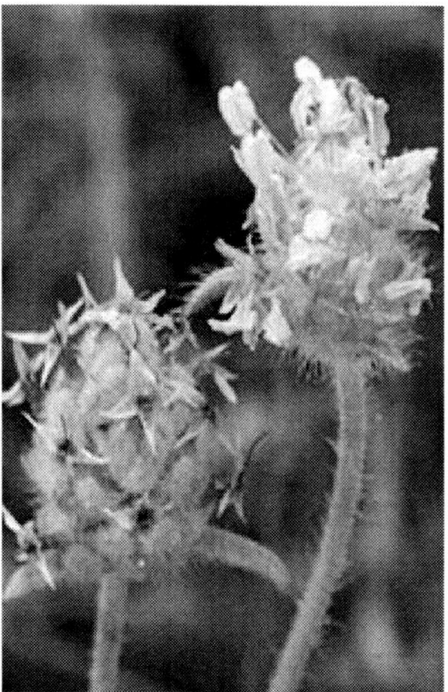

Plantago Psyllium
Plantain Family
Part Used: Whole or ground seeds, gathered in summer and autumn when ripe
Habitat: Europe; Jersey; northern Africa; southern Asia.

Also known as: Fleaseed; Ispaghula; Psyllion; Psyllios; Psyillium Plantain; Plantego; Plaintain; Psyllium Husks

Dosage: 60 - 240 grains

- Do not take with other supplements - forms an indigestible mass.
- Do not take within 1 hour of other prescriptions since it interferes with absorption.
- Do not use in presence of low blood sugar.
- **Do not use during pregnancy - stimulates lower pelvis.**
- Must take with a lot of water to prevent intestinal blockage.

Primary Uses:
Bowels - promotes regularity
Constipation
Fiber
Hemorrhoids
Inflammation, internal & tissue - soothes
Intestines - cleanses & lubricates
Laxative
Stool softener

Secondary Uses:
Bronchitis - loosens phlegm & coats mucous membranes
Colitis
Crohn's disease
Diarrhea - retains waters
High cholesterol
Irritable Bowel Syndrome
Pneumonia - loosens phlegm & coats mucous membranes
Ulcers, stomach

Other Possible Uses:
Dysentery
Heart disease
Throat, sore

- Lowers levels of blood glucose and cholesterol by preventing absorption in intestines.
- Does not cause cramps.

Queen of the Meadow

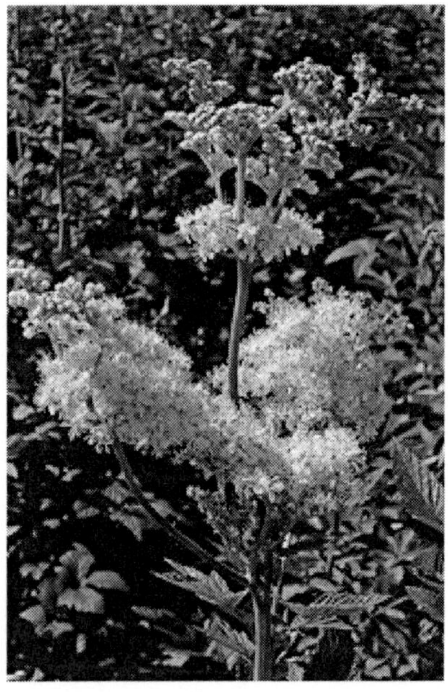

Spiraea Ulmaria
Rose Family
Part Used: Herb
Habitat: Worldwide.

Also known as: Bridewort; Dolloff; Lady of the Meadow; Meadowsweet; Meadsweet

Dosage: 30 grains

Primary Uses:
Astringent
Bladder infections (one of the best)
Diarrhea, especially children
Diuretic - tea
Fever - infusion of fresh tops
Inflammation, internal - soothes
Kidney infections (one of the best)
Stomach disorders
Gas

Secondary Uses:
Detox
Dropsy
Flu
Perspiration - produces, infusion of fresh tops

Other Possible Uses:
Antacid
Arthritis
Gas

- Infusion: 1 ounce to 1pint water in wineglassful doses.
- Used in mead and herbal beers.

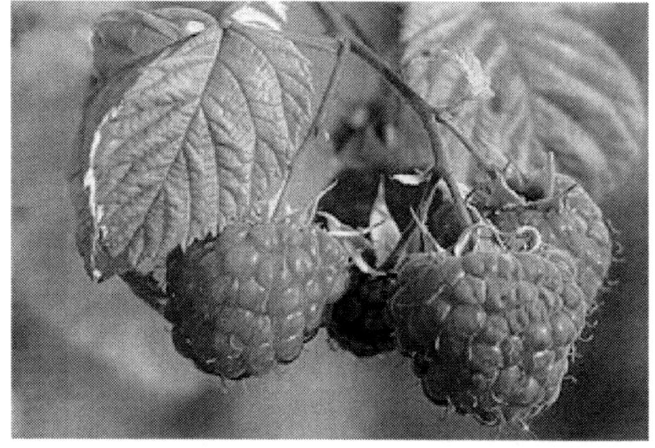

Raspberry

Rubus Idaeus
Rose Family
Part Used: Leaf
Habitat: Europe; Great Britain.

Also known as: Bramble of Mount Ida; European Raspberry; Hindberry; Raspbis; Red Raspberry

Dosage: 1 tsp. to 1 cup water

- **May be unsafe to use during first few months of pregnancy as it induces labor and may cause miscarriage.**

Primary Uses:
Antibiotic
Appetite suppressant
Astringent
Bones - promotes healthy
Cramps
Detox
Diarrhea, especially in children
Hot flashes
Kidney
Labor - induces
Liver
Menstrual bleeding, excessive
Morning sickness - with peppermint (also for diarrhea)
Nails - promotes healthy nails
Premenstrual Syndrome - relieves cramps and flow
Skin - promotes healthy skin
Spasm, intestinal
Stimulant
Teeth - promotes healthy teeth
Uterus - strengthens

Secondary Uses:
AIDS
Bedwetting
HIV
Labor pains
Lungs, inflammation
Mother's milk

External Uses:
Burns - poultice with slippery elm, stops oozing
Canker Sores
Sore mouth - gargle
Sore throat - gargle
Ulcers - wash
Wounds – wash

- **The tea is wonderful against morning sickness, but keep in mind that it induces labor, so do not overdo it.**
- Added to feed of pregnant goats to help with a safe, trouble-free delivery.
- Relaxes tight uterine muscles and tightens relaxed uterine muscles.
- **Very controversial herb - use caution during pregnancy for morning sickness. Ginger tea is much safer.**

Red Clover

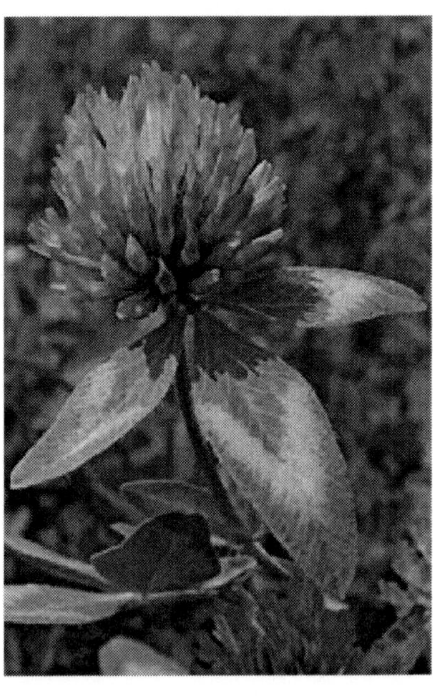

Trifolium pratense
Legume Family
Part Used: Blossoms
Habitat: Britain; central and northern Asia; Europe; United States.

Also known as: Honey; Honeystalks; Purple Clover; Shamrock; Three-Leaved Grass; Trefoil; Trifoil

Dosage: 30 - 60 grains

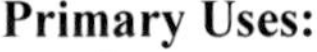

Primary Uses:
AIDS
Antibiotic
Antispasmodic - extract
Appetite suppressant
Arthritis
Blood cleanser
Bronchitis - infusion
Detox - extract
Gout
HIV
Lungs, inflamed
Muscle relaxer
Relaxant
Sedative
Tuberculosis
Whooping cough - infusion

Secondary Uses:
Cancer preventative
Coughs
Expectorant
Kidney
Liver

Other Possible Uses:
Chest
Eczema
Hepatitis
Mono

External Uses:
Athlete's foot
Cancerous growths - poultice
Eczema
Psoriasis
Wounds, mucus

- Infusion: 1 ounce to 1 pint water.

Rhubarb

Rheum Rhaponticum
Buckwheat Family
Parts Used: Roots, Stems
Habitat: China; cultivated worldwide.

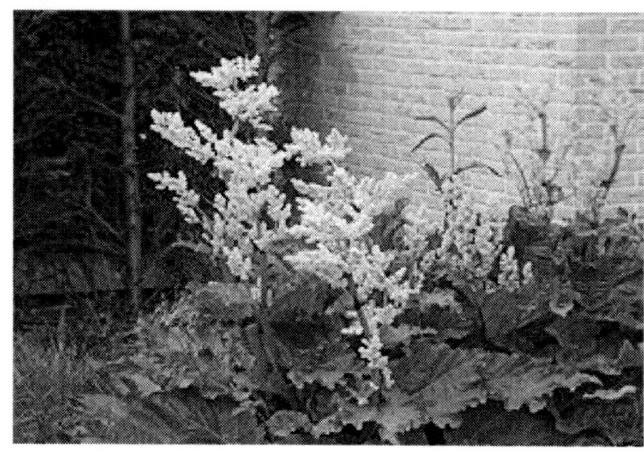

Also known as: Bastard Rhubarb; Cultivated Lucern; Garden Rhubarb; Purple Medicle; Sweet Round-leaved Dock

Dosage: 5 - 10 grains

- **May be fatal in some cases - use caution.**
- Do not use often.
- **Do not use if pregnant.**
- Keep away from open wounds - will burn them.

Primary Uses:
Antibiotic
Astringent
Constipation
Diarrhea
Headache
Hemorrhoids
Liver disorders
Purgative
Stomachic
Ulcers, duodenal

Secondary Uses:
Bowels
Colon disorders
Spleen disorders
Worms, especially thread worms

Other Possible Uses:
Dysentery
Fever
Hemorrhaging

External Uses:
Ulcer

Rose Hips

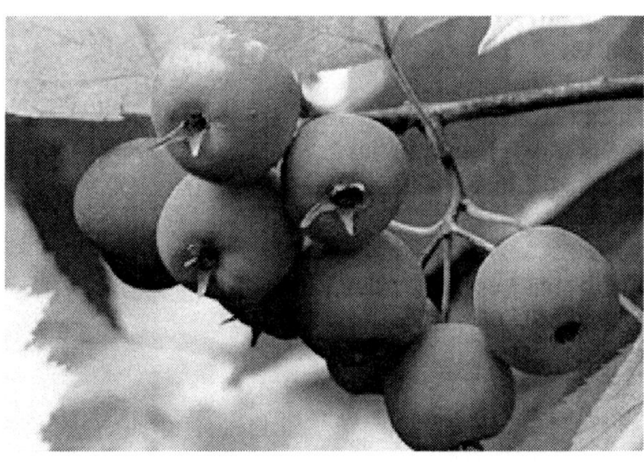

Rosaceae
Rose Family
Part Used: Hips
Habitat: Middle East; worldwide.

Also known as: Dog Brier; Dog Rose; Hip Tree; Rose Haws; Wild Brier

Dosage: 30 - 60 grains

Primary Uses:
Bladder problems
Diarrhea - tea
Infections, all
Stress

Secondary Uses:
Diuretic
Headache

- Rose hip wine:
    - 3 pounds rose hips 3 pounds sugar
    - 1 gallon boiling water
    - Wash rose hips and cut in half. Place in a large bowl and pour water over them. Stir with a wooden, not metal, spoon Cover bowl and leave for 2 weeks. Strain liquid into another bowl and add sugar, stirring until dissolved. Cover and leave for 5 days, stirring daily. Bottle, loosely corked, and store in a cool dark place for 6 months. The corks may be pushed down once the wine has stopped fermenting.

- The syrup of rose is added to water in the Middle East for stomach upset and fainting.
- Extremely high in vitamin C.

Rosemary

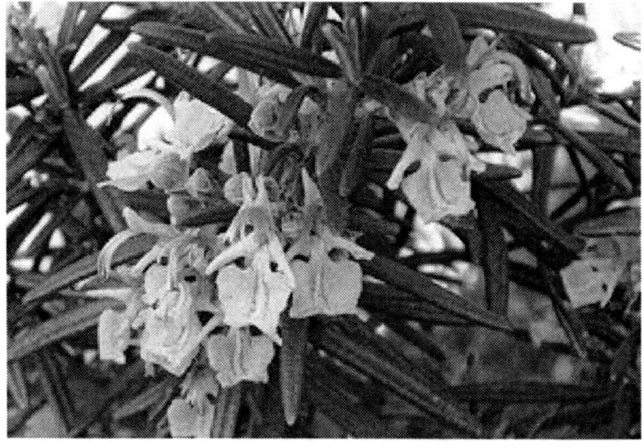

Rosmarinus officinalis
Mint Family
Parts Used: Herb, Root
Habitat: Worldwide.

Also known as: Compass Plant; Compass Weed; Dew of the Sea; Elf Leaf; Guardrobe; Incensier; Polar Plant; Sea Dew

Dosage: 30 - 60 grains

- Oil irritates stomach, causes heartburn and may damage kidneys.
- Large amounts of oil cause deep coma, spasms, vomiting, gastroenteritis, uterine bleeding, kidney irritation, pulmonary edema (fluid in the lungs) and death.
- Rosemary baths in the evening may cause insomnia. They are stimulating.
- **Do not use during pregnancy - high dosage may cause miscarriage.**
- Do not use in presence of epilepsy - the camphor in the herb may aggravate seizures.
- Avoid if have heavy menstrual periods - may aggravate.

Primary Uses:
Antioxidant
Astringent
Circulation, especially brain
Colds - tea
Colic - tea
Cramps
Depression, nervous - tea
Gas - oil
Headaches - oil & tea
Liver toxicity
Nerves
Perspiration - produces
Stimulant
Stomachic - oil
Tonic

Secondary Uses:
Alzheimer's
Antibacterial
Anti-fungal, yeast
Antiseptic
Antispasmodic
Asthma - smoke with coltsfoot
Cancer
Digestion
Diuretic
Dizziness
Heart - stimulant with wine
High blood pressure
High cholesterol
Indigestion
Irritable Bowel Syndrome - relieves cramps, spasms & bloating
Menstrual cramps

Other Possible Uses:
Anti periodic
Appetite stimulant
Tumors

External Uses:
Anti fungal
Bad breath
Baldness, premature - infusion with borax
Brain function – oil, inhale fumes (stimulates)
Bruises - bath
Circulation
Cuts
Dandruff - with olive oil
Eczema - bath
Gout - steeped in water then distilled, for hands & feet
Low blood pressure - bath
Migraines - oil rubbed on temples
Pain - bath
Rheumatism - bath
Skin - bath
Sprains - bath
Strains
Varicose veins - bath
Wounds

- For fresh breath, the distilled water of rosemary flowers may be drunk first thing in the morning and last thing before bed. For sweet breath, add cloves, mace, cinnamon and anise.
- Traditionally burned in hospitals with juniper berries to prevent the spread of infection.
- Stimulates the release of bile.

Sage

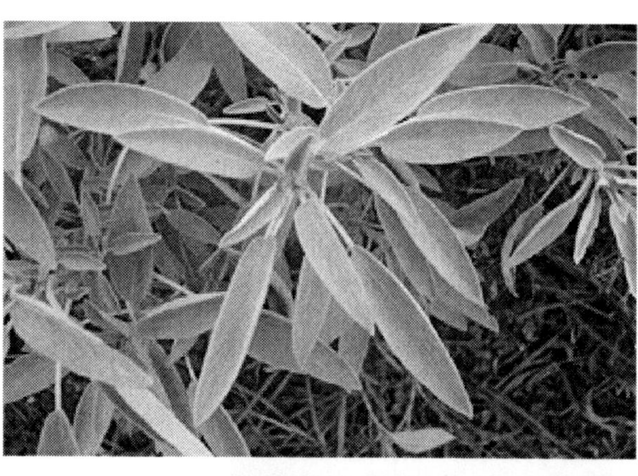

Salvia officinalis
Mint Family
Part Used: Leaves, Whole Herb
Habitat: Northern shores of the Mediterranean to the east side of the Adriatic.

Also known as: Broad Leaved White Sage; Garden Sage; Narrow Leaved White Sage; Red Sage; Sawge; White Sage

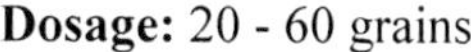

Dosage: 20 - 60 grains

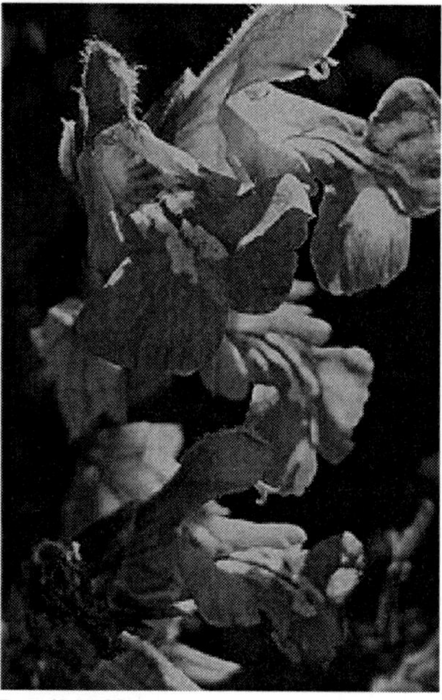

- Do not use in presence of seizure disorders.
- Do not use two weeks at a time consecutively.
- **Do not use during pregnancy or while nursing.**

Primary Uses:
Astringent
Colds - tea
Detox - tea
Digestion, slow & weak - tea
Expectorant
Fever - tea
Gas
Headache, nervous - strong infusion
Hemorrhaging, lungs & stomach - tea
Kidney - tea
Liver, complaints & biliousness - tea
Measles - tea
Memory
Nervous diseases - tea
Pain, joint - tea
Perspiration, excessive - tea
Stimulant
Tonic
Typhoid fever - tea
Weak stomach

Secondary Uses:
Bronchitis
Estrogen deficiency
Hot flashes
Night sweats
Tonsillitis

Other Possible Uses:
Catarrh
Cramps, menstrual
Indigestion
Mother's milk - dries
Nasal problems

External Uses:
Athlete's foot
Bleeding gums - gargle
Canker sores - wash & gargle
Douche
Hair growth - rinse
Itchy skin
Muscles, sore - bath
Sores - infusion
Teeth - brush
Throat, inflamed & sore - gargle
Tired feet - bath
Tonsils, sore - gargle

Sarsaparilla

Smilax officinalis
Smilax Family
Part Used: Root
Habitat: Central America; Costa Rica.

Also known as: Bamboo Brier; China Root; Chinese Root; Red Bearded Sarsaparilla; Small Spikenard; Smilax Medica; Vera Cruz; Wild Sasp

Dosage: 30 - 60 grains

- Tinctures made with alcohol are not effective - the active constituents are soluble in water but not in alcohol.
- Large doses may produce gastrointestinal irritation.
- **Do not use during pregnancy or while nursing.**
- Increases the rate at which the body absorbs digitalis compounds.
- Increases the rate at which the body expels tranquilizers.

Primary Uses:
Arthritis
Detox
Diuretic
Fever
Gout, pain - stimulates excretion of uric acid
Impotence
Perspiration - produces profuse
Rheumatism - swelling & soreness
Urinary tract disorders
Sex drive - men & women
Sexually transmitted diseases
Syphilis

Other Possible Uses:
Frigidity
Infertility
Metabolism - stimulates
Nervous system disorders
Premenstrual Syndrome

Secondary Uses:
Catarrh
Chest complaints
Colds - syrup
Coughs - syrup
Eczema
Energy - increases
Erectile dysfunction
Hormones - regulates
Psoriasis
Radiation exposure - protects against

External Uses:
Eczema
Hives
Leprosy
Psoriasis
Ringworm
Shingles - wash
Skin diseases
Ulcers, indolent - wash
Wounds – heals

- Will not relieve an acute gout attack but helps prevent attacks from occurring when taken over a period of several weeks or months.
- Stimulates production of testosterone.

Sassafras

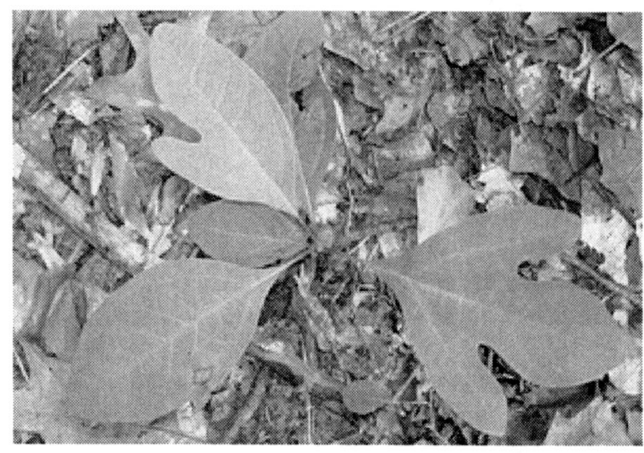

Sassafras officinale
Laurel Family
Part Used: Root
Habitat: Eastern United States; Mexico.

Also known as: Laurus Sassafras; Sassafrax

Dosage: 30 - 60 grains

- **Abortive - Do not use during pregnancy.**
- May cause liver cancer.
- Do not use oil internally - causes narcotic poisoning. (Fatal - death by widespread fatty degeneration of the heart, liver and kidneys, depression of circulation, followed by centric paralysis of respiration.)

Primary Uses:
Blood cleanser
Detox
Gonorrhea
Lungs - damage from tobacco, prevents & removes
Perspiration - produces
Rheumatism - with sarsaparilla
Skin disease - purifies blood, with sarsaparilla
Stimulant
Syphilis - with sarsaparilla
Tobacco - helps quit

Secondary Uses:
Poison ivy - tea

Other Possible Uses:
Antispasmodic
Arthritis
Colds - preventative
Diuretic
Gout
Muscle relaxant

External Uses:
Eyes - wash in rosewater (stand for four hours then filter)
Moth repellent
Poison ivy

- One tsp. of oil in one man produced vomiting, dilated pupils, stupor and collapse.
- My family has used the root tea for generations with no adverse effects. Make sure to use only the root - do not get too close to the stem, as it is poisonous. So are the leaves.

Saw Palmetto

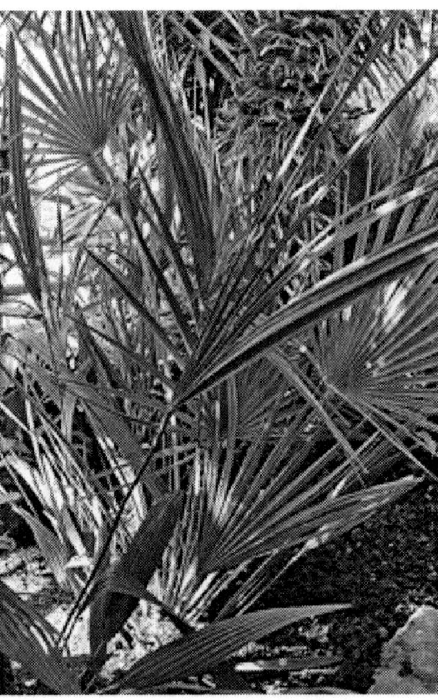

Serenoa serrulata
Palm Family
Part Used: Berries
Habitat: Atlantic coast from South Carolina to Florida; southern California.

Also known as: American Dwarf Palm Tree; Cabbage Palm; Sabal; Sabal Serenoa; Serrulata

Dosage: 5 - 20 grains

- Do not use with hormone replacement therapy or oral contraceptives.
- **Avoid even handling this herb during pregnancy or when attempting to become pregnant - the berries have both estrogenic and anti-estrogenic properties.**
- Fresh berries frequently cause diarrhea.
- Take with food to avoid stomach upset.
- Do not make tea from the dried herb. The medicinal oils do not dissolve in water.

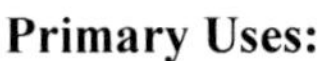

Primary Uses:
Antiseptic, urinary
Aphrodisiac - with damiana
Appetite stimulant
Diuretic
Genitals, irritation
Hormone regulation
Prostate, enlarged, cancer & all problems - takes 6-8 weeks to notice effects

Secondary Uses:
AIDS, weight loss
Anti-inflammatory
Asthma
Breast enlargement
Bronchitis, chronic (sedative)
Colds
Expectorant
HIV, weight loss
Menopause - reduces growth of facial & body hair without interfering with hormone levels
Muscle building

External Uses:
Genitals, irritation

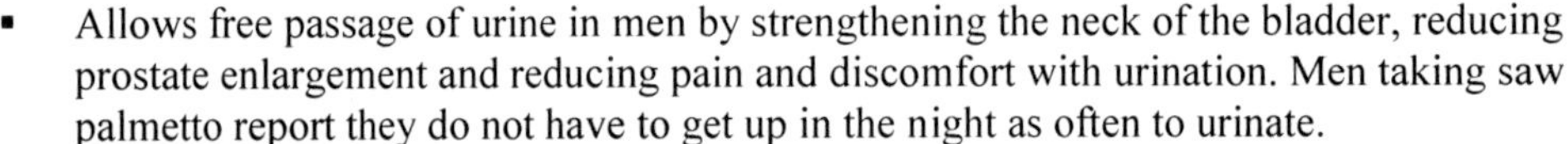

- Allows free passage of urine in men by strengthening the neck of the bladder, reducing prostate enlargement and reducing pain and discomfort with urination. Men taking saw palmetto report they do not have to get up in the night as often to urinate.
- Slows cell division in prostate tissue by reducing availability of dihydrotestosterone. Does not reduce testosterone. Also reduces swelling caused by accumulation of fluid in prostate tissue faster than prescriptions.
- Stimulates deposit of proteins in muscle tissue and counteracts severe weight loss in chronic diseases.

Schizandra

Drosera schizandra
Magnolia/Schizandra Family
Part Used: Berries
Habitat: China; Japan; Korea; Russia.

Also known as: Gumishi; Magnolia Vine; Schisandra; Schisandra Fruit; Wu-wei-zi

Dosage: 400 - 450 mg per day

- Increases flow of bile. Avoid in presence of gallstones or bile duct blockage.
- **Do not use during pregnancy - stimulates uterus and induces labor.**
- Avoid in presence of high blood pressure, peptic ulcers and epilepsy.

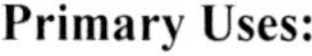

Primary Uses:
Aphrodisiac
Depression
Fatigue
Impotency
Liver, all diseases, cancer, chemical damage, hepatitis, AIDS, inflammation, tissue destruction, etc.
Sedative
Stamina, sexual
Stress, especially emotional
Tonic - youth
Adrenal gland health
Blood pressure - normalizes
Blood sugar - normalizes
Dizziness
Headache
High cholesterol
Insomnia
Restless Leg Syndrome
Sweating, excessive
Vision, acuity & field of vision

Secondary Uses:
Adaptogen - increases the body's resistance to stress & disease

Other Possible Uses:
Cancer, skin, after chemical injury
Morphine overdose - antidote

- Helps rebuild cells by energizing RNA and DNA.
- Helps protect the heart muscle during chemotherapy treatments using Doxorubicin without interfering with Doxorubicin's effect on cancer cells.
- Helps speed recovery from liver surgery.

Scullcap

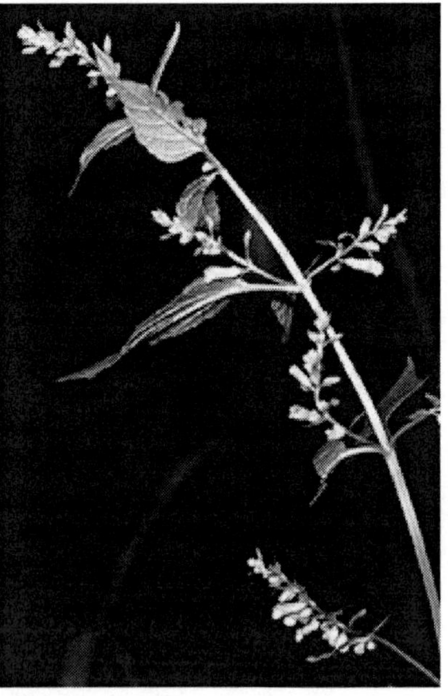

Scutellaria lateriflora
Mint Family
Part Used: Herb
Habitat: Worldwide in temperate and tropical mountain regions; most abundant in the United States.

Also known as: Greater Scullcap; Helmet Flower; Hoodwort; Mad-Dog Scullcap; Madweed; Virginian Scullcap. Other Scullcaps known as Greater Scullcap; Helmet Flower; Hoodwort

Dosage: 15 grains

- Do not overdose - produces dizziness, confusion, erratic pulse, giddiness, stupor and twitching of the limbs. (Similar to epilepsy.)

Primary Uses:
Alcoholism
Antispasmodic
Anxiety
Calms the body
Cardiovascular disease
Circulation
Convulsions (one of the best)
Cramps, menstrual
Depression
Epilepsy
Headaches, nervous & from coughing (one of the best)
Heart - strengthens
Hiccups, severe
Hydrophobia
Hyperactivity
Hysteria
Insomnia
Irritability
Migraines
Muscle cramps, spasms, pain & tension
Nerves, all disorders
Nervous excitement - soothes
Nervous weakness
Pain, muscular
Restlessness
Rheumatism
Rickets
Seizures
Sleep - induces
Stress

Secondary Uses:
Barbiturate addiction
D.T.'s
Drug withdrawal
Fatigue
Rabies

Other Possible Uses:
Antibacterial
Anti periodic
Depressant, central nervous system
Tonic
Uterine relaxer

Senna

Cassia Acutifolia
Legume Family
Parts Used: Dried leaves, Pods
Habitat: Arabia; Egypt; Nubia; Sennar.

Also known as: Alexandrian Senna; Cassia Aethiopica; Cassia Angustifolia; Cassia Lanceolata; Cassia Lenitiva; Cassia Officinales; Cassia Senna; East Indian Senna; Egyptian Senna; Nubian Senna; Senna Acutifolia

Dosage: 30 - 120 grains

- **Do not use while nursing** - causes purging in the infant.
- May cause griping and nausea - do not take alone. Mix with cloves, ginger, cinnamon, fennel, etc.
- Steep instead of boil to lessen pain.
- **Do not use during pregnancy.**
- Do not use in presence of intestinal inflammation.

Primary Uses:
Constipation
Purgative - very powerful

Secondary Uses:
Detox
Stimulant - slight
Worms (used following wormwood)

External Uses:
Pimples
Skin diseases

Shepherd's Purse

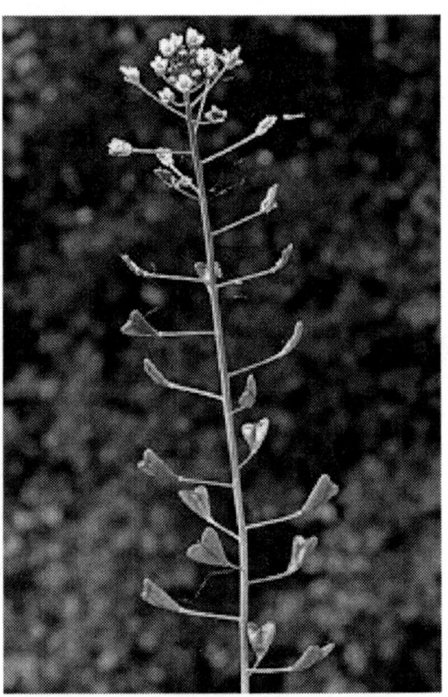

Capsella bursa-pastoris
Cabbage Family
Parts Used: Aerial Parts
Habitat: Worldwide, outside the tropics.

Also known as: Blindweed; Case-weed; Casewort; Clappedepouch; Lady's Purse; Mother's Heart; Pepper and Salt; Pick Pocket; Pick Purse; Poor Man's Parmacettie; Rattle Pouches; Sanguinary; Shepherd's Bag; Shepherd's Scrip; Shepherd's Sprout; Toy-wort; Witch's Pouches

Dosage: 30 grains

- **Do not take during pregnancy - causes uterine contractions and coagulates blood.**
- Causes blood clotting.

Primary Uses:
Blood vessels - contracts
Diarrhea, chronic - astringent
Diuretic
Hemorrhaging, all, especially kidneys & uterus - dried & infused (one of the best)
Menstruation, excessive
Scurvy
Tissues - contracts
Womb, parturition during childbirth - causes contractions

Secondary Uses:
Bladder, catarrh & abscesses
Dropsy - with couch grass
Dysentery
Hemorrhoids
Kidney complaints - with couch grass
Urine, mucus - relieves
Uterus - tones after childbirth & helps return to normal size

Other Possible Uses:
Bedwetting, children
Fever
Stimulant

External Uses:
Bruises - bruised herb
Ear pain - juice drops
Nosebleed - juice on cotton
Rheumatism
Strains - bruised herb
Wounds, bleeding - stops

Slippery Elm

Ulmus fulva
Elm Family
Parts Used: Inner bark of trunk and branches, collected in the spring
Habitat: Canada; United States.

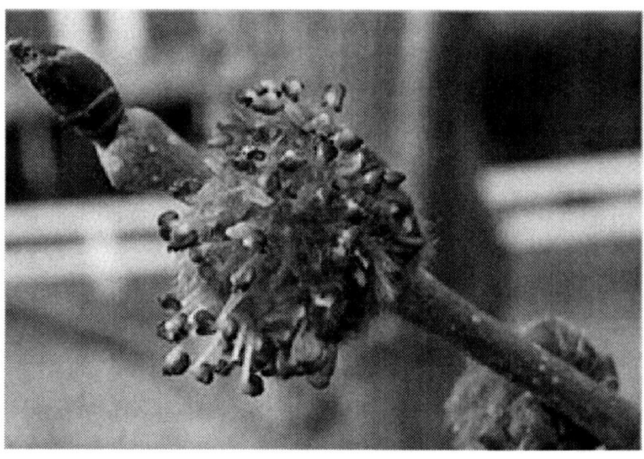

Also known as: Indian Elm; Moose Elm; Red Elm; Sunset Elm

Dosage: 60 grains

- May interfere with absorption of medications if taken at the same time.

Primary Uses:
Bowel inflammation
Bronchitis - drink (one of the best)
Colitis - drink 3x a day
Coughs - compound (one of the best)
Diarrhea
Diuretic
Expectorant
Gas - drink 3x a day
Hemorrhaging, all
Inflammation, internal & tissue
Lungs, bleeding - drink 3x a day
Nutritive
Sleep - drink at night
Stomach inflammation - drink
Tapeworm - with oil of male fern
Throat, sore
Typhoid Fever - compound
Urinary disease & inflammation

Secondary Uses:
Colds
Crohn's disease
Digestive irritation
Dysentery
Flu
Food poisoning
Heart - drink
Indigestion
Laxative for children without pain
Ulcers, peptic
Vomiting, pain after

External Uses:
Abscesses - poultice (one of the best)
Boils - poultice
Bowel inflammation - enema
Burns - poultice
Constipation - enema
Douche
Eruptions - poultice (one of the best)
Gangrene - poultice with infusion of wormwood & charcoal
Inflammation - poultice
Pain - poultice with vinegar & wheat bran
Skin, itchy, inflamed, irritated, dry & diseases - poultice
Swelling - poultice
Ulcers - poultice (one of the best)
Wounds - poultice (one of the best)

- Poultice: Mix slippery elm with hot water until desired consistency. Spread on cotton cloth and cover part of body desired. If using on hair (such as arm or chest), use olive oil first.
- Drink: Mix slippery elm into cold water to form a paste. Pour boiling water into paste until it turns to liquid. Flavor with cinnamon or other flavoring if desired.
- Compound: Mix 1ounce (or more if desired) bark with a pinch of cayenne and a slice of lemon. Infuse. Let stand for 25 minutes. Use 1 pint per day in small frequent doses.
- Slippery elm makes a great gruel with as much nutrition as oatmeal. It is good for infants and invalids, especially when other foods fail.
- Native Americans soak the inner bark in water and put on wounds. It dries into a natural bandage. They also wrap it around pieces of meat to prevent spoilage.

- Slippery elm soothes and heals any part of the body it touches.
- No upper limit on dosage. Safe and used as a food product.

Solomon's Seal

Polygonatum multiflorum
Lily Family
Part Used: Root
Habitat: England; Ireland; northern Europe; Siberia.

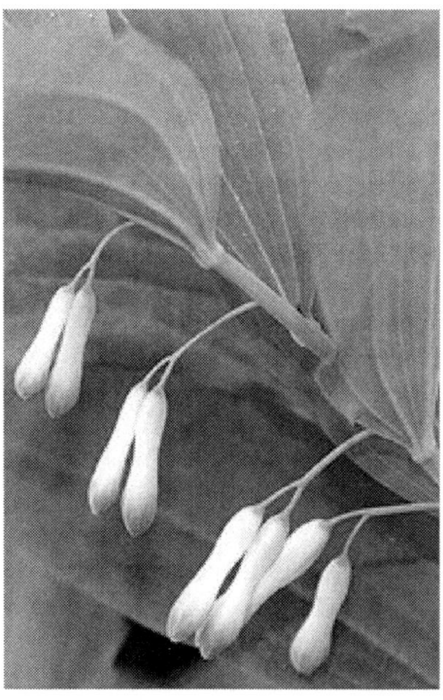

Also known as: Dropberry; Lady's Seals; St. Mary's Seal; Sealroot; Sealwort

Dosage: 30 - 60 grains

- The berries cause vomiting - do not use.
- The leaves cause nausea - do not use.

Primary Uses:
Astringent
Bowel inflammation - infusion
Broken bones - decoction with wine (one of the best)
Dysentery, chronic - infusion
Inflammation
Lungs - bleeding, infusion
Stomach inflammation - infusion
Tonic
Women's problems

Secondary Uses:
Expectorant
Pain, internal

External Uses:
Black eye - bruised root with cream or lard
Bruises - poultice
Complexion - distilled water of root
Cuts
Hemorrhoids - wash
Inflammation - poultice
Piles - wash or poultice
Poison ivy - wash (one of the best)
Sneezing - induces, snuff
Sores
Tumors - poultice
Wounds

St. John's Wort

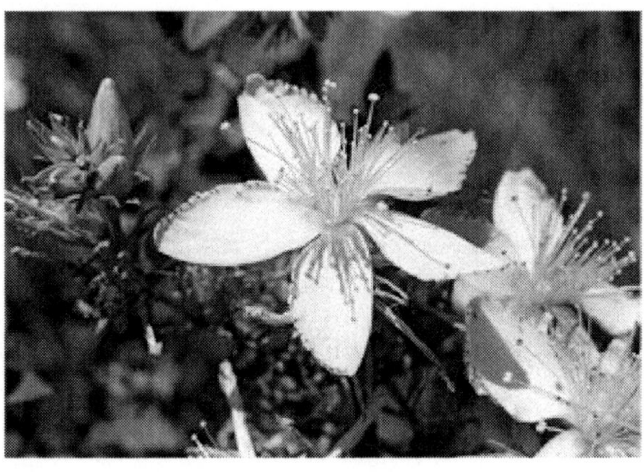

Hypericum perforatum
St. John's Wort Family
Parts Used: Petals gathered at Midsummer (traditional), Entire plant (modern)
Habitat: Asia; Britain; Europe.

Also known as: Amber; Goatweed; Herba John; Hypericum; Klamath Weed; Scare Devil; Sol Terrestis; Tipton Weed

Dosage: 60 grains

- **Do not use during pregnancy.**
- Causes photosensitivity - stay out of the sun and tanning beds during use.
- Decreases effectiveness of oral contraceptives, protease inhibitors (for HIV), Elavil, Coumadin, etc.
- Avoid use with monoamine oxidase inhibitors.
- May cause severe episodes of high blood pressure when combined with tyramine (found in aged cheeses, red wine, chocolate, etc.)
- Intensifies effects of anesthesia.
- Do not use with Tramadol (for pain) or Sumatriptum (for migraines) or other medications that influence serotonin levels - may cause Serotonin Syndrome, which may be life threatening.

Primary Uses:
Anxiety
Astringent
Bedwetting - infusion
Bladder problems
Breasts, caked
Crohn's disease
Depression, nervous
Diarrhea
Diuretic
Dysentery
Emotional problems
Expectorant
Gastrointestinal problems
Headache, tension & fever
Hemorrhoids
Hysteria
Insomnia
Irritable Bowel Syndrome - overnight (used in Europe)
Jaundice
Melancholia
Nerves
Pain
Spitting blood - with knotgrass
Urine - suppresses
Worms, especially intestinal

Secondary Uses:
AIDS
Bronchitis
Cramps
Gout - tea
Herpes
HIV
Liver
Muscle relaxer
Tranquilizer - mild
Ulcers
Viral infections
Vomiting

Other Possible Uses:
Abortive
Uterine cramping

External Uses:
Antibacterial
Back pain
Boils
Breasts, caked
Bruises

Burns, pain - ointment (heals 3x faster)
Cancer - used with sunlight
Cold sores (Herpes Simplex 1)
Cuts
Staph sores & infection
Swelling
Throat - bread, strengthens (good for singers)
Tumors
Wounds – compress

- Oils and tinctures should be dark red from the hypericin constituent.
- Relaxes blood vessels, increases circulation and counteracts blood vessel constriction caused by inflammatory chemicals such as histamines, etc.

Tea Tree

Melaleuca leucadendron
Clove Family
Parts Used: Oil, Leaves, Small Branches
Habitat: East Indies; tropical Australia.

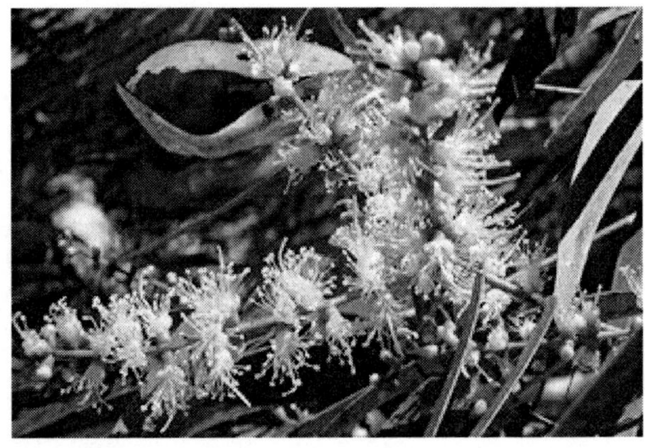

Also known as: Cajuput; Swamp Tea Tree; White Tea Tree; White Wood

Dosage: No recommended dosage.

- If irritation occurs on skin, dilute with vitamin E oil or primrose oil. If this does not help, discontinue.
- **The oil is dangerous when used internally. Causes nerve damage.**
- Oil is irritating to genitals.
- Test oil on inner arm - if it turns red or becomes inflamed, do not use.
- Do not use if allergic to thyme or celery.

Primary Uses:
Perspiration - produces
Pulse - increases
Stimulant
Warming

Secondary Uses:
Antiseptic
Antispasmodic
Bronchitis
Cystitis
Expectorant
Laryngitis
Worms, especially round worms

Other Possible Uses:
Rheumatism

External Uses:
Acne - oil
Athlete's foot - oil
Bites, insect & spider - oil
Colds - gargle with water
Cold sores - oil
Cuts - disinfects, oil
Cystitis - oil
Dermatitis - oil
Disinfectant - oil
E. coli, on skin - kills 90%
Fungal infections - oil
Herpes - oil
Psoriasis - oil
Scabies - oil
Skin affections - oil
Staphylococcus, on skin - kills 90%
Throat, sore - gargle with water
Vaginitis - oil
Warts - oil
Wounds - disinfects, oil
Yeast infections - douche with water

Thyme

Thymus vulgaris
Mint Family
Part Used: Leaves
Habitat: Worldwide in temperate climates.

Also known as: Common Thyme; Creeping Thyme; French Thyme; Garden Thyme; Mountain Thyme

Dosage: 30 - 60 grains

- **Do not use during pregnancy - abortive.**
- Do not use in presence of duodenal ulcer.
- May cause abdominal contractions.
- Discontinue using in bath if inflammation develops.
- Using as toothpaste or mouthwash may cause swollen tongue or cracks in corners of mouth - dilute or discontinue.
- **Oil used internally may cause vomiting, dizziness, convulsions, coma, cardiac arrest and respiratory arrest.**

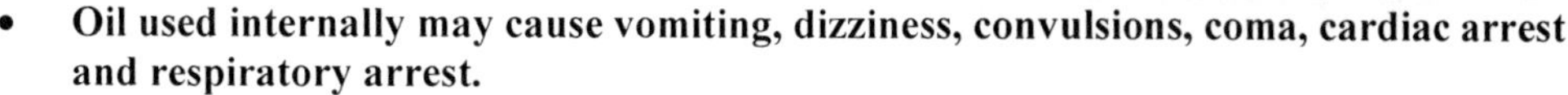

- May suppress normal thyroid activity in medicinal doses.

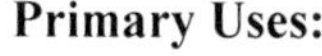

Primary Uses:
Antiseptic
Antispasmodic - steam or oil
Asthma
Colds - tea
Coughs - steam or oil
Croup
Epilepsy
Fever - tea
Flu
Gas - tea
Headache - tea
High cholesterol
Liver disease
Mucus - reduces
Respiratory problems, chronic
Sinusitis
Throat, sore
Tonic
Whooping cough - fresh, pounded with syrup

Secondary Uses:
Brain
Diuretic
Emmenagogue
Gout
Gums
Internal disorders
Labor - induces
Melancholia
Mouth
Nerves
Pain in the hips
Paralysis
Parasites - oil
Perspiration - produces, tea
Stimulant
Stomachic
Teeth
Urination - soothes
Worms, intestinal

External Uses:
Anti fungal
Antiseptic
Athlete's foot - extract
Crabs, lice, etc. - extract
Deodorant
Disinfectant
Genital pain - douche
Germicide
Gout
Mouthwash
Pain, aches
Parasites
Rheumatism - bath
Scalp, itching
Shingles - ointment
Sore throat - gargle

Sprains - bath
Swelling - ointment & bath
Teeth - oil, paste or mouthwash
Warts - ointment
Yeast infection

- Cough syrup:
    - ½ ounce dried thyme
    - ¼ ounce dried sage
    - ¼ ounce dried chamomile
    - 2 tsp. fennel seeds
    - 1 tsp. anise seed
    - 20 cloves
    - 2 garlic cloves
    - Pinch cayenne and ground ginger
    - 3 ¾ cup water
    - 1 pound honey

- Primary ingredient in some popular mouthwashes.
- Used to preserve meat.

Turmeric

Curcuma longa
Ginger Family
Parts Used: Root, Rhizome
Habitat: Bengal; China; Java; southern Asia.

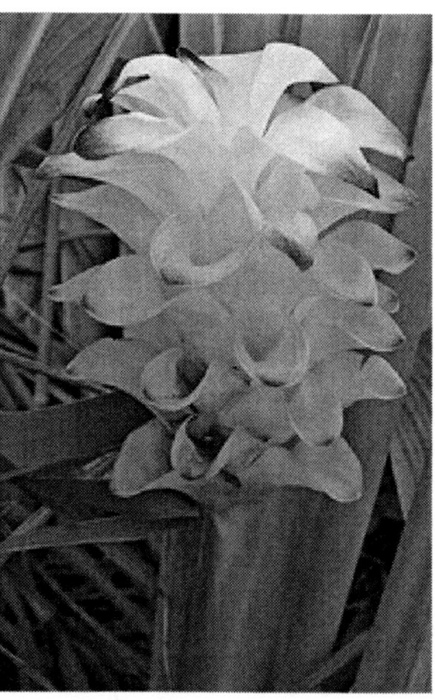

Also known as: Curcuma; Gauri; Haldi; Indian Saffron; Olena; You Jin

Dosage: 15 - 30 grains

- Avoid large quantities.
- Interferes with proper functioning of breast cancer chemotherapy.
- Do not use in presence of bile duct blockage, blood clotting disorders, peptic ulcers or gallbladder problems.
- May reduce fertility. (Does so in lab animals.)
- May inhibit blood clotting.

Primary Uses:
Antibacterial
Antibiotic
Anti-inflammatory
Arthritis
Gallbladder disease & stones
High cholesterol
Indigestion
Jaundice
Liver, cirrhosis - protects & detox
Stimulant

Secondary Uses:
AIDS
Arteriosclerosis
Blood clots - preventative
Bursitis
Cancer - kills several types of cancer cells*
Carpal Tunnel Syndrome
Cataracts - preventative (over many years)
Endometriosis
Heart attack, tissue damage
High blood pressure
HIV
Obesity
Pain, shoulder

Other Possible Uses:
Colic
Cramps, menstrual
Nightmares
Stomach disorders

External Uses:
Arthritis
Halitosis
Periodontal disease - prevents

*Inhibits spread of melanoma to lungs and keeps tumors from spreading throughout the body. Aids in recovery by stimulating the immune system and may even prevent cancer from smoking, colorectal, etc.

- Used as yellow dye.
- Prevents HIV from advancing into AIDS (protease inhibitor).
- Accelerates liver detox and prevents alcohol and toxins from being converted into harmful forms in the liver. Also reverses liver damage from iron absorption.
- Relaxes blood vessels.

Valerian

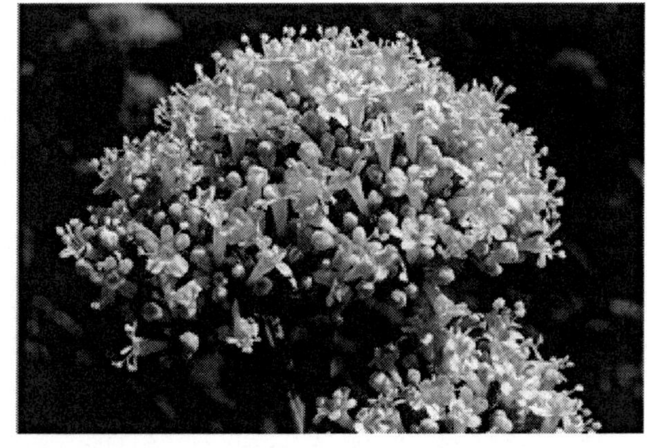

Valeriana officinalis
Valerian Family
Parts Used: Leaf, Root dried below 105° f
Habitat: Europe; northern Asia.

Also known as: All-Heal; Amantilla; Bloody Butcher; Capon's Tail; Capon's Trailer; Cat's Valerian; English Valerian; Fragrant Valerian; Garden Heliotrope; Great Wild Valerian; Phu; Red Valerian; St. George's Herb; Sete Wele; Setewale; Setwall; Setwell; Vandal Root

Dosage: 10 - 15 grains

- **Do not use during pregnancy - abortive.**
- Overdose produces weak heartbeat, pain in the head, heaviness and stupor.
- May impair attention. Do not take with narcotics, muscle relaxers, sleep medications or tranquilizers.
- Do not use more than 2 consecutive weeks.
- Do not use with alcohol - ever.
- If used over a long period of time, may cause withdrawal symptoms if stopped abruptly.
- May increase effects of barbiturates and tranquilizers.
- Large doses produce giddiness, light-headedness and liver toxicity.
- Do not use with Valium, Elavil, sedatives or antidepressants.
- Do not give to children under 12 years old.

Primary Uses:
Anticonvulsant
Antispasmodic
Anxiety
Cerebral stimulant & excitant
Circulation
Colic
Cramps, menstrual
Epilepsy
Fatigue
Gas
Headaches
Hypochondria
Hysteria
Indigestion, nervous
Insomnia, especially chronic
Irritable Bowel Syndrome - stops spasms
Irritability
Muscle tension & cramps
Nerves & nervous overstrain
Pain
Panic, especially night attacks
Sedative, nervous system
Sleep
Stimulant
Stress
Tension
Ulcers

Secondary Uses:
Aphrodisiac
High blood pressure
Menopause related problems
Palpitations, heart
Restless Leg Syndrome
Stomach cramps

Other Possible Uses:
Alcoholism
Anti-aphrodisiac
Asthma
Child behavioral disorders
Colds
Hiccups
Indigestion

Psychedelic	Tonic

- Non-addictive.

Violet

Viola odorata
Violet Family
Parts Used: Dried flowers and leaves, fresh whole plant
Habitat: Temperate and tropical regions of the world.

Also known as: Blue Violet; Sweet Violet

Flowers:
Dosage: 30 - 60 grains

Primary Uses:
Expectorant - fresh flowers
Whooping cough

Secondary Uses:
Colds
Eyes, inflammation - syrup
Headache - syrup
Hoarseness
Inflammation - syrup
Insomnia - syrup
Laxative - slight, syrup
Lungs, all diseases - dried flowers
Tumors - dissolves & heals

Other Possible Uses:
Detox
Epilepsy - syrup
Jaundice - syrup
Pleurisy - syrup

Leaves:
Dosage: 30 - 60 grains

Primary Uses:
Cancer & pain, throat
Cancer of tongue - infusion (½ drank & ½ applied hot) - see recipe
Detox (one of the best)
Tumors - dissolves & heals
Whooping cough

Other Possible Uses:
Fever - drink
Jaundice
Laxative

Secondary Uses:
Antiseptic
Colds
Eyes, inflammation - leaves & flowery tops, decoction
Hoarseness

External Uses:
Bruises
Coolant - plaster
Inflammation - plaster or poultice
Swelling - plaster or poultice

Roots:
Dosage: 30 grains

Other Possible Uses:
Emetic - strong, produces great vomiting
Nervous affections
Purgative - strong

- Infusion: Taken cold. 2-½ ounces leaves, wash, place in jar and pour 1 pint boiling water over them. Cover and let stand 12 hours or until water is green. Strain. Take one wineglassful every 2 hours until gone. Make this fresh every day. Any leftovers should be thrown away.

White Oak

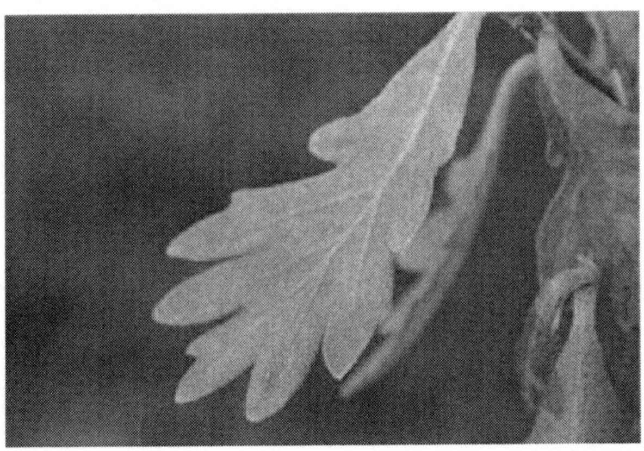

Quercus alba
Beech Family
Part Used: Bark
Habitat: Eastern United States.

Also known as: Quebec Oak

Dosage: 15 grains

- Contains high levels of tannins.

Primary Uses:
Antiseptic
Bladder problems
Fever
Gallstones
Goiter
Hemorrhoids
Kidneys
Premenstrual Syndrome
Varicose veins

Secondary Uses:
Bleeding from mouth - stops
Diarrhea
Hemorrhaging
Mucous discharge
Nosebleed
Vomiting

External Uses:
Antiseptic
Astringent
Burns
Douche
Piles - ointment
Poison ivy
Sores, badly healing - poultice
Sore throat - gargle
Stings, bee
Teeth
Ulcers - poultice
Varicose veins
Wounds

White Willow

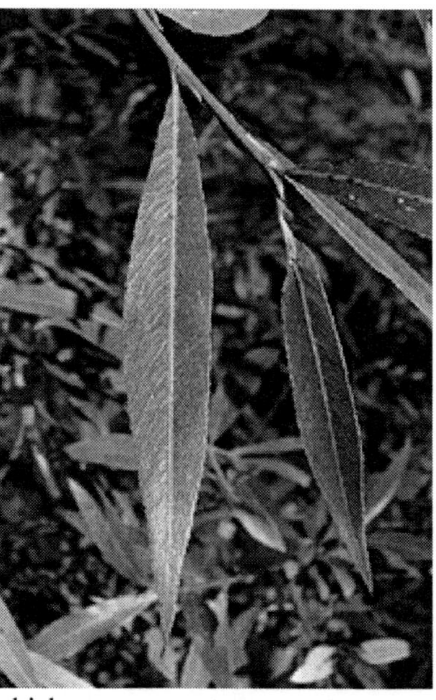

Salix alba
Willow Family
Part Used: Bark of 2 - 5 year old trees in spring
Habitat: Central and southern Europe.

Also known as: European Willow; Osier; Pussy Willow; Saille; Salieyn Willow; Saugh Tree; Tree of Enchantment; Witchs' Aspirin; With; Withy

Dosage: 15 - 30 grains

- Contains salacin.*
- Do not take with aspirin, ibuprofen or naproxen - may cause stomach bleeding.
- High doses produce: stomach upset, nausea and tinnitus (ringing in the ears).
- Do not use in presence of peptic ulcers or tinnitus.
- Do not give to children under 16 for any cold, flu or chicken pox symptoms - may cause Reye's Syndrome. (Metabolized differently than commercial aspirin, but they are very close.)
- May diminish sex drive and interest.
- Do not use if have allergic reaction to aspirin.
- **Do not use during pregnancy or while nursing.**

Primary Uses:
Anesthetic
Antiperiodic
Arthritis
Backache - 1 week+
Diarrhea, chronic
Digestion
Dysentery
Fever
Headaches (one of the best)
Pain, especially inflammation
Tonic
Toothaches
Worms

Secondary Uses:
Colds
Osteoporosis - 1 week+
Rheumatism

External Uses:
Acne - sap
Bruises - compress
Cuts - compress
Dandruff - infusion of bark & leaves
Deodorant - with borax
Pimples - wash
Skin – bath

*White willow is used instead of aspirin without a lot of the side effects. However, it has salacin (or salicylic acid), the same ingredient as aspirin, so do not use it if allergic to aspirin or on any medication prohibiting use of aspirin. (Aspirin was originally made from this.)

- Works longer than commercial aspirin without aspirin's side effects.
- Has no effect on platelets and does not increase bleeding or irritate the stomach lining like commercial aspirin does.

Witch Hazel

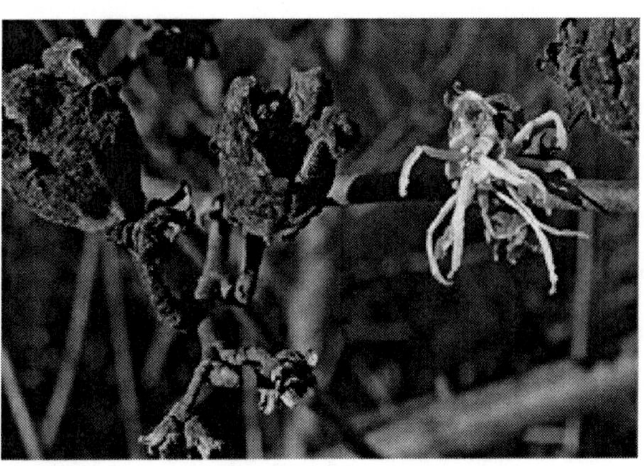

Hamamelis virginiana
Witch Hazel Family
Parts Used: Leaves, Bark
Habitat: Canada; eastern United States.

Also known as: Hamamelist; Spotted Alder; Snapping Hazelnut; Winterbloom

Dosage: 30 - 60 grains

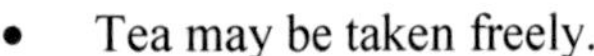

- Tea may be taken freely.
- Do not use commercial or other alcohol-based witch hazel water - it has no good effect from the herb and may even be dangerous when used internally.
- May cause stomach upset, nausea, vomiting and constipation.

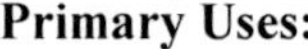

Primary Uses:
Abortion, debilitated state after & problems arising from
Bowel complaints - speedy relief
Diarrhea, acute not chronic - bark tea is one of best
Dysentery
Gleet
Hemorrhaging, internal & external (all)
Pain
Piles, bleeding - tea (excellent & fast)
Sedative
Stomach bleeding - tea
Tonic

Secondary Uses:
Menstruation, excessive
Varicose veins

External Uses:
Astringent - cooling
Breasts, sore
Bruises
Bug bites - liquid on cotton (fast relief)
Burns
Cold sores
Cuts
Eczema
Eyelid inflammation - diluted extract
Eyewash
Feet, tired
Gums & teeth, sore
Hemorrhoids
Inflammation
Insect bites
Itching
Joints, sore
Muscles, sore
Pain
Periodontal disease - gargle or mouthwash
Phlebitis
Piles
Poison ivy
Rectal surgery, discomfort - relief
Skin tonic
Sore throat
Sunburn - anti-inflammatory effect
Swelling
Tumors, painful
Vaginal surgery, discomfort - relief
Vaginitis - douche
Varicose veins - applied on bandage & kept moist
Wounds, small
Wrinkles – smoothes

- Mixed with cucumber juice for enlarged pores.
- Great for shaving nicks.

Wormwood

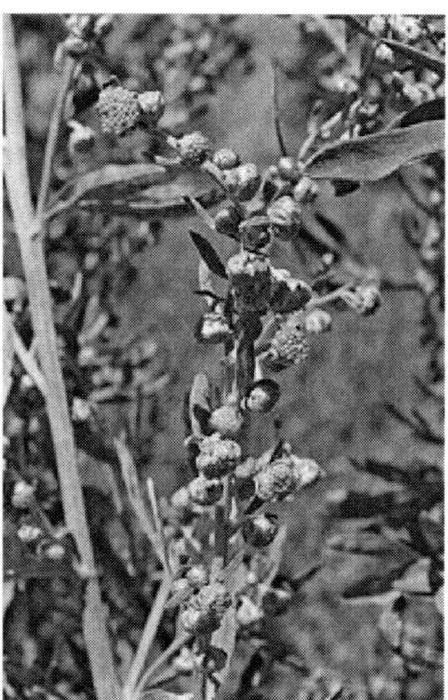

Artemisia Absinthium
Composite Family
Parts Used: Whole Herb
Habitat: Europe; Siberia; United States.

Also known as: Absinthe; Crown for a King; Green Ginger; Old Woman

Dosage: 15 - 20 grains

- Habit forming.
- **Do not use during pregnancy - may cause spontaneous abortion.**
- Overdose will irritate stomach and increase heart action.
- As a tea, it contains too low a concentration of thejone to be as dangerous as absinthe, but is still something to be used carefully, if at all.
- Tea made too strong will have the opposite effect.

Primary Uses:
Fever - reduces
Gout - 1 ounce in 1 pint brandy steeped 6 weeks, 1 tbls. before meals & bed
Stomachic - increases activity
Tonic
Worms - expels (intestinal), flowers, dried & powdered. Especially for roundworms. May be combined with black walnut for parasites.

Secondary Uses:
Appetite stimulant - tops of plant fresh infusion
Diarrhea
Digestion - improves, tops of plant fresh infusion
Jaundice - promotes bile
Liver disease
Mental restorative
Nerve tonic
Sedative - mild
Sickness after meals
Stimulant

Other Possible Uses:
Diabetes
Female complaints
Gas
Migraine
Spinal irritation
Tonsil inflammation

External Uses:
Bruises - poultice
Fallen arches & bad ankles - rub
Fleas - repels on cats & dogs, stuffed in their beds
Inflammation - poultice
Insect repellent - clothes, pantry, etc.
Moth repellent - clothes, pantry, etc.
Rheumatism - local anesthetic, oil
Sprains - poultice
Swelling - poultice

- Absinthium stimulates the cerebral hemispheres and is a direct stimulant of the cerebral cortex. Too much causes epileptic like convulsions and giddiness. Absinthe itself is illegal in many countries as it is very addictive and dangerous. Use wormwood with care. As always, respect the herb and don't abuse it.

Yarrow

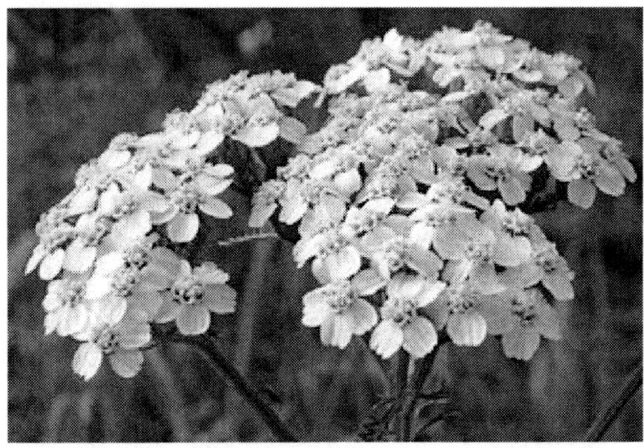

Achillea millfolium
Composite Family
Parts Used: Flowers, Leaves, Stems
Habitat: Worldwide.

Also known as: Achilhea; Arrowroot; Bad Man's Plaything; Bloodwort; Carpenter's Weed; Deathflower; Devil's Nettle; Devil's Plaything; Eerie; Field Hops; Gearwe; Hundred Leaved Grass; Knight's Milfoil; Knyghten; Lady's Mantle; Milfoil; Militaris; Military Herb; Millefolium; Noble Yarrow; Nose Bleed; Old Man's Pepper; Sanguinary; Seven Year's Love; Snake's Grass; Soldier's Woundwort; Stanch Griss; Staunchweed; Tansy; Thousand Weed; Woundwort; Yarroway; Yewr

Dosage: 30 - 60 grains

- **Do not use during pregnancy - uterine stimulant.**
- Avoid in presence of heavy periods.
- May increase sensitivity to sun.
- Clean wounds well before applying this herb - stops bleeding so fast that may trap dirt, bacteria and other contaminants.
- Increases production of bile and may intensify gallstone pain.
- May stop sperm production (alcohol extracts). It does in mice - not tested in humans.

Primary Uses:
Anti inflammatory, intestinal & female reproductive tract
Astringent
Bleeding piles
Blood clotting - improves
Chicken pox
Colds, severe - tea with cayenne
Colitis
Diarrhea
Diuretic
Fever, severe - tea with cayenne
Flu
Hemorrhaging, all
Kidney disorders
Measles - tea with cayenne
Menstrual disorders, cramping, pain
Perspiration - produces, tea
Smallpox
Stimulant
Stomach, cramps
Tonic
Ulcers
Viral infections

Secondary Uses:
Abortive
Digestion - improves
Gas
Heart, nervous conditions
Hemorrhoids
Liver
Rheumatism
Sedative - mild
Vision, blurred

Other Possible Uses:
Bones
Bronchitis
Emmenagogue
Gas
Hair
Heartbeat - slows
High blood pressure
Indigestion
Leucorrhoea

External Uses:
Baldness - wash
Blackheads - infusion
Bleeding - stops
Boils

Bruises
Cuts
Douche
Inflammation
Pain
Toothache - wash
Vaginal problems
Venereal disease
Wounds - poultice
Wound discharge

Yerba Santa

Eriodictyon glutinosum
Waterleaf Family
Part Used: Leaves
Habitat: California; northern Mexico.

Also known as: Bear's Weed; Bearweed; Consumptive's Weed; Gum Bush; Holy Herb; Mountain Balm; Sacred Herb

Dosage: 15 - 60 grains

Primary Uses:
Asthma - tea & smoke, or chew leaves
Bladder irritation
Bronchial irritation
Expectorant
Hay fever
Hemorrhoids
Laryngitis
Tonic

Secondary Uses:
Coughs, nagging
Diarrhea
Phlegm

Other Possible Uses:
Arthritis
Colds
Detox
Gonorrhea
Headaches - tea
Hoarseness
Rheumatism
Syphilis
Throat irritation
Venereal disease
Vomiting

External Uses:
Headache - compress
Herbal tobacco
Pain - poultice
Swelling - poultice
Thirst - chew

Yucca

Yucca Filamentosa, Yucca Brevifolia, Yucca Glauca
Agave Family
Part Used: Root
Habitat: Central America; North America; West Indies.

Also known as: Adam's Needle; Mojave Yucca; Needle Palm; Our Lord's Candle; Soapweed; Spanish Bayonet; Spanish Dagger; Spanish Needle

Dosage: No recommended dosage.

- Long-term use may disrupt absorption of the fat-soluble vitamins. (A, D, E, K, etc.)

Primary Uses:
Arthritis, pain & inflammation
Osteoporosis
Rheumatism, pain & inflammation

Secondary Uses:
Detox
Inflammatory disorders

Other Possible Uses:
Cancer
Pain
Tumors

- Flowers are used in perfume.
- Used for baskets, mats, shoes and paper for weather stripping.
- Fruit may be eaten raw or cooked.
- Roots used for cleaning hair and washing clothes, especially wool.

Part Two

Disorders Listed Alphabetically

When using this section of the book, it is best to refer back to Part One to make sure the correct herbs are used for the situation at hand. Check on side and other effects of each herb before using it to treat any disorder.

If there is any specific information associated with a particular herb pertaining to the disorder it is listed with, it is listed in this manner:

Herb name - how used (any specific type of disorder or information)

Abscesses:

Primary:
Dandelion

Other Possible:
Garlic
Lobelia

External:
Chickweed - poultice in muslin (one of the best)
Comfrey
Fenugreek - poultice
Slippery Elm - poultice

Acne:

Primary:
Oregon Grape
Primrose

Secondary:
Mistletoe

External:
Black Walnut
Echinacea - cream
Golden Seal
Hawthorne
Lady's Mantle
Lavender
Oregon Grape
Tea Tree - oil
Willow - sap
Yarrow (black heads)

Adaptogen:

Secondary:
Schizandra

Addictions:

Primary:
Kudzu - one of the best (alcohol)
Scullcap (alcohol)

Secondary:
Golden Seal - with cayenne (alcohol)
Parsley (alcohol)
Scullcap (barbiturates)

Other Possible:
Alfalfa - stops (narcotics)

Adrenal:

Primary:
Borage - tonic
Licorice (promotes function)

Secondary:
Schizandra (health)

Other Possible:
Milk Thistle (disorders)

Afterbirth:

Other Possible:
Angelica (expels)

Age Spots:

Primary:
Raspberry Leaf
Red Clover

AIDS:

Primary:
Red Clover

Secondary:
Astragalus
Cat's Claw
Cinnamon
Licorice
Pau D'Arco
Raspberry Leaf
St. Johns Wort
Saw Palmetto (weight loss)
Turmeric

Alcoholism:

Primary:
Ginger (gastritis)
Hops (D.T.'s)
Kudzu (removes cravings)
Lady's Slipper (D.T.'s)
Milk Thistle (liver problems)
Scullcap

Secondary:
Cayenne
Golden Seal - with cayenne
Parsley
Primrose

Other Possible:
Alfalfa (helps stop)
Angelica (stops cravings)
Valerian

Allergies:

Primary:
Ma Huang
Nettles (all allergies)
Secondary:
Chamomile
Ginger (especially food allergies)
Gingko Biloba (inflammation)
Licorice
Pau D'Arco
Peppermint (food allergies)

(Allergies, cont'd.)

External:
Eucalyptus
Oregon Grape (rashes)

Alzheimer's:

Primary:
Gingko Biloba (symptoms)

Secondary:
Gotu Kola
Hawthorne
Rosemary

Anaphrodesiac:

Secondary:
Chaste Tree

Other Possible:
Valerian

Anemia:

Primary:
Dandelion
Fenugreek
Nettles

Secondary:
Angelica (cold hands & feet)
Dong Quai

Other Possible:
Alfalfa
Bilberry - fruit
Hawthorne

Anesthetic:

Primary:
White Willow

External:
Allspice - ointment & bath
Kava Kava (local)
Oregon Grape (local)
Peppermint - oil (local)

Angina:

Secondary:
Angelica
Astragalus - one of the best (pain)

Anorexia:

Primary:
Caraway

Antacid:

Secondary:
Chickweed

Other Possible:
Queen of the Meadow

Analgesic:

Secondary:
Kava Kava

External:
Cloves
Kava Kava
Myrrh

Anti -abortive:

Secondary:
Catnip

Other Possible:
Cramp Bark

Antibacterial:

Primary:
Agrimony
Chamomile
Golden Seal
Pau D'Arco
Turmeric

Secondary:
Garlic
Rosemary

Other Possible:
Elecampane (bactericide)
Peppermint
Scullcap

External:
Agrimony
Aloe Vera
Astragalus
Barberry - on skin (kills)
Chamomile
Lavender
Myrrh - gargle
St. John's Wort
Yarrow

Antibiotic:

Primary:
Echinacea
Garlic
Golden Seal
Raspberry Leaf
Red Clover
Rhubarb
Turmeric

Secondary:
Barberry - one of the best

Other Possible:
Balm of Gilead
Horseradish

Anticonvulsant:

Primary:
Catnip
Chamomile (infantile)
Cramp Bark
Lobelia
Scullcap - one of the best
Valerian

Secondary:
Blue Vervain
Lady's Mantle
Lavender
Mistletoe

Other Possible:
Anise (safe)
Chickweed
Ginger
Golden Seal

Antidotes:

Belladonna (opium, chloroform, calabur bean)
Coffee (hemlock)
Feverfew (opium)
Frankincense (hemlock)
Mustard - with castor oil (emetic - hemlock)
Nettles - seeds (hemlock, henbane, nightshade)
Tannic Acid (hemlock)
Zinc - emetic (hemlock)

These are not a substitute for hospitalization - poisons are not something to mess around with - seek professional help immediately!

Anti-fungal:

Primary:
Garlic
Pau D'Arco

Secondary:
Alfalfa
Cinnamon
Rosemary (yeast)

External:
Aloe Vera
Black Walnut
Chamomile - with vinegar
Cloves
Echinacea - cream
Garlic (inhibits)
Lavender
Pau D'Arco
Rosemary
Tea Tree Oil (infections)
Thyme

Anti-Histamine

Primary:
Chamomile

Anti-Inflammatory:

Primary:

Arrowroot (internal & bowel)
Buchu, bladder - infusion
Butchers Broom (all, especially kidneys)
Catnip
Cat's Claw
Chamomile
Chickweed (internal)
Coltsfoot, internal - soothes
Comfrey, internal - soothes
Corn Silk - soothes (internal, bladder & kidneys)
Couch Grass - soothes (internal, bladder & kidneys)
Devil's Claw
Echinacea
Golden Seal (especially chronic colon)
Juniper
Licorice - soothes (internal tissue)
Marshmallow (mucous membranes & stomach)
Mullein (all internal)
Pleurisy (lungs)
Psyllium - soothes (internal tissue)
Queen of the Meadow - soothes (internal)
Slippery Elm (urinary, internal, tissue, bowel & stomach)
Solomon's Seal (stomach & bowel)
Turmeric
Yarrow
Yucca (arthritis & rheumatism)

Secondary:

Alfalfa (bladder)
Aloe
Bilberry - fruit, leaves & bark
Blessed Thistle
Blue Cohosh (uterine)
Borage (internal & tissue)
Buchu (prostate)
Cayenne
Cranberry (internal)
Ginger
Gingko Biloba (allergies)
Gravel Root (prostate)
Horseradish (urinary)
Horsetail
Pau D'Arco
Saw Palmetto
St. John's Wort
Violet - flowers - syrup (especially eyes)
Yucca (disorders)

Other Possible:

Barley Grass
Bilberry - fruit (bowel)
Boneset
Buchu (colon, gums, mucous membranes, sinus & vaginal)
Horseradish (lungs)
Milk Thistle - soothes (internal)
Wormwood (tonsil)

External:

Agrimony- gargle (throat)
Aloe
Arnica (joint)
Bayberry - gargle (throat, chronic)
Blue Vervain - poultice
Catnip - poultice
Cat's Claw
Chamomile (skin)
Chickweed - poultice
Cloves
Elder - flowers (general), cold tea (eyes)
Elder - leaves - juice (eyes), ointment (soothing)
Fennel - ointment
Ginger
Hops - with Chamomile - one of the best
Horsetail - juice
Lady's Mantle
Lobelia - poultice
Marshmallow - warm poultice
Myrrh (mouth & throat)
Sage - gargle (throat)
Slippery Elm - poultice
Solomon's Seal
Violet - leaves - plaster or poultice (especially eyes)
Witch Hazel - poultice
Wormwood - poultice
Yarrow

Anti-Irritant:

Secondary:

Cayenne

Antimicrobial:

Secondary:

Catnip
Fennel

External:

Cloves

Antioxidant:

Primary:

Cat's Claw
Gingko Biloba
Green Tea
Rosemary

Secondary:

Chamomile

Antiperiodic:

Primary:

White Willow

Other Possible:

Rosemary
Scullcap

Antiseptic:

Primary:

Barberry
Bilberry - fruit (urinary tract)
Echinacea (blood)
Garlic
Horseradish
Saw Palmetto (urinary)
Thyme
White Oak

Secondary:

Angelica
Buchu
Lavender
Violet - leaves

Other Possible:

Anise
Elecampane
Tea Tree

External:

Balm of Gilead
Barberry
Cinnamon
Cloves (powerful)
Elecampane (pain during surgery - Do not attempt this - only a qualified physician should perform surgeries)
Eucalyptus
Garlic
Lavender
Myrrh
Peppermint - oil
Tea Tree - oil
Thyme
White Oak

Antispasmodic:

Primary:
Belladonna (asthma & colic)
Blue Cohosh (muscular)
Catnip
Cramp Bark
Lady's Slipper
Lobelia
Ma Huang (bronchial)
Mistletoe
Peppermint
Red Clover - extract
Scullcap
Thyme - oil or steam
Valerian

Secondary:
Angelica (stomach & bowels)
Blue Vervain
Chamomile
Ginger
Licorice (muscular, decreases spasms)
Pleurisy
Rosemary
Tea Tree

Other Possible:
Coltsfoot
Honeysuckle
Lavender
Mullein
Pennyroyal
Sassafras

Anti-Viral:

Primary:
Cat's Claw
Echinacea
Garlic
Yarrow

Secondary:
Licorice
St. John's Wort

Other Possible:
Hyssop

(Anti-Viral, cont'd.)

External:
Aloe Vera

Anxiety:

Primary:
Chamomile
Hops
Kava Kava
Lady's Slipper
Lavender
Passion Flower
Scullcap
St. John's Wort
Valerian

Secondary:
Damiana

Other Possible:
Bilberry - fruit
Primrose

Aphrodisiac:

Primary:
Damiana
Echinacea
Gotu Kola
Saw Palmetto - with Damiana
Schizandra

Secondary:
Cinnamon
Parsley
Valerian

Other Possible:
Anise

Appetite Stimulant:

Primary:
Blessed Thistle
Caraway (powerful)
Catnip
Centuary
Chamomile
Cayenne
Dandelion
Fennel
Ginger
Golden Seal
Gotu Kola
Hops
Lavender
Myrrh
Peppermint

Secondary:
Alfalfa - tea
Boneset
Devil's Claw
Horehound (especially with flu)
Hyssop
Parsley
Wormwood

Other Possible:
Juniper - small doses
Lady's Mantle

Appetite Suppressant:

Primary:
Guarana
Raspberry Leaf
Red Clover

Secondary:
Ma Huang

Arthritis:
See also Rheumatism & Inflammation

Primary:
Alfalfa
Cat's Claw (all forms)
Chamomile
Devil's Claw (very good)
Feverfew
Garlic
Nettles
Red Clover
Sarsaparilla
Turmeric
White Willow
Yucca (pain & inflammation)

Secondary:
Agrimony
Astragalus (rheumatoid)
Bilberry (rheumatoid)
Black Cohosh
Blue Cohosh
Burdock - tea
Cayenne
Comfrey (rheumatoid)
Feverfew (rheumatoid pain)
Ginger
Hawthorne (rheumatoid & osteoporosis)
Horsetail
Primrose
White Willow (rheumatoid & osteoporosis)

Other Possible:
Black Pepper
Butcher's Broom (swelling & pain)
Horseradish
Licorice (pain)
Queen of the Meadow
Sassafras
Yerba Santa

External:
Arnica
Bladderwrack - bruised leaves
Cayenne
Eucalyptus
Fennel - oil
Rosemary (rheumatoid)
Turmeric

Asthma:

Primary:

Black Cohosh
Blue Vervain
Chamomile
Coltsfoot - tea or smoke
Comfrey
Cramp Bark (antispasmodic)
Elecampane
Fennel
Garlic - syrup
Green Tea
Honeysuckle - syrup (nervous)
Horehound
Lobelia
Ma Huang
Marshmallow
Mullein - smoke
Nettles - juice with honey or sugar
Thyme
Yerba Santa - tea, chew leaves or smoke

Secondary:

Anise (spasmodic)
Burdock
Cat's Claw
Cayenne
Elder - berries - hot wine
Fenugreek
Ginger
Gingko Biloba
Horseradish - with honey
Hyssop - green tops boiled in soup
Licorice
Primrose
Rosemary - with coltsfoot

Other Possible:

Alfalfa
Juniper
Valerian

External:

Nettles - smoke leaves
Rosemary - smoke with coltsfoot

Astringent:

Primary:

Agrimony
Bayberry
Bilberry - fruit
Black Walnut - bark
Comfrey
Elder - flower water
Eyebright
Gravel Root
Horsetail
Lady's Mantle
Mullein
Myrrh
Nettles
Queen of the Meadow
Raspberry Leaf
Rhubarb
Rosemary
Sage
Solomon's Seal
St. John's Wort
White Willow
Yarrow

Secondary:

Hawthorne
Primrose

Other Possible:

Dragon's Blood
Elecampane
Ginger
Poke - root

External:

Barberry
Blue Vervain
Cinnamon
Comfrey
Myrrh
Oregon Grape
White Oak
Witch Hazel (cooling)

Athlete's Foot:

External:

Agrimony
Alfalfa
Black Walnut
Pau D'Arco
Red Clover
Sage
Tea Tree - oil
Thyme

Backache:

Primary:

Chamomile
White Willow

External:

Belladonna - poultice
St. John's Wort

Bad Breath (Halitosis):

Primary:

Alfalfa
Anise
Cloves - chewed whole
Myrrh - rubbed on gums (disease)
Parsley
Peppermint
Rosemary
Turmeric

Secondary:

Hawthorne

Balding:

See also Hair

External:

Burdock
Nettles
Rosemary - infusion with borax (premature)
Yarrow - wash

Bedwetting:

Primary:

Agrimony
Corn Silk - with agrimony
Damiana
Kava Kava
Parsley
St. John's Wort

Secondary:

Horsetail
Raspberry Leaf

Other Possible:

Shepherd's Purse (children)

Bed Sores:

External:

Comfrey
Myrrh

Bee Stings:

External:

Arrowroot
Comfrey
Lavender
Parsley - poultice
White Oak

Biliousness:

Primary:

Barberry
Milk Thistle (increases bile)

Black Eye:

External:
Solomon's Seal - bruised root with cream

Bladder:

Primary:
Agrimony
Blue Vervain (relieves)
Buchu
Butcher's Broom (infection & tonic)
Chamomile
Corn Silk (irritation & inflammation)
Couch Grass (disease & inflammation)
Cranberry (prevents bacteria)
Gotu Kola (infection)
Hops (infection)
Horsetail (problems)
Juniper - oil (disease)
Marshmallow (infection & pain)
Mistletoe (disorders)
Nettles (disorders)
Parsley
Queen of the Meadow - one of the best
Rose Hips
Slippery Elm (disease & inflammation)
St. John's Wort
White Oak
Yerba Santa (irritation)

Secondary:
Alfalfa (inflammation)
Angelica (infection)
Astragalus (infection)
Cat's Claw
Garlic (infection)
Gravel Root (infection)
Horsetail (problems)
Kava Kava (infection)
Shepherd's Purse (catarrh & abscesses)

Other Possible:
Horseradish (infection)
Licorice (ailments)

Bleeding:
See Blood Clotting

Bleeding Gums:

External:
Alfalfa
Sage – gargle

Bleeding Piles:

Primary:
Yarrow

Blemishes:

External:
Elder - flower water
Hawthorne

Blood Cleanser:
See Detox

Blood Clotting:

Primary:
Dong Quai (dissolves clots)
Garlic (preventative)
Hawthorne (strengthens vessels)
Shepherd's purse (all blood clotting)

Secondary:
Agrimony (promotes clotting)
Blessed Thistle (stops bleeding)
Butcher's Broom (reduces, constricts vessels)
Turmeric (prevents clotting)

Other Possible:
Gingko Biloba (prevents clotting)

External:
Agrimony
Yarrow - one of the best

Blood Sugar:

Secondary:
Schizandra (normalizes)

Blurred Vision:

Secondary:
Yarrow

Boils:

Primary:
Dandelion

External:
Black Walnut
Blessed Thistle
Burdock
Comfrey
Dandelion
Dong Quai
Echinacea
Elder - flower water
Fenugreek
Golden Seal
Hops
Horehound (dissolves)
Pau D'Arco
Slippery Elm
St. John's Wort
Tea Tree – oil

Bones:

Primary:
Comfrey - one of the best (broken)
Horsetail (strengthens weak or broken)
Raspberry Leaf (healthy)
Solomon's Seal - decoction with wine - one of the best

Other Possible:
Butcher's Broom (broken)
Yarrow

External:
Comfrey (broken)

Bowels:

Primary:
Cascara Sagrada (tones)
Mullein - with milk (bleeding)
Nettles
Psyllium (promotes regularity)
Slippery Elm (inflammation)
Solomon's Seal (inflammation)
Witch Hazel (speedy, all complaints)

Secondary:
Chickweed
Oregon Grape (sluggish)
Rhubarb

Other Possible:
Bilberry - fruit (inflammation)

External:
Slippery Elm - enema - see page

Brain Function:

Primary:
Blessed Thistle
Chamomile (fatigue)
Gingko Biloba
Hops (fatigue & overuse)
Rosemary (circulation)

Secondary:
Parsley
Thyme

External:
Rosemary - inhale scent of oil

Breasts:

Primary:
Dandelion (tumors)
Primrose (tenderness)
St. John's Wort (caked)

Secondary:
Saw Palmetto (enlarges)

Other Possible:
Lady's Mantle (sagging)

External:
Lady's Mantle (sagging)
St. John's Wort (caked)
Tea Tree - oil (mastitis)
Witch Hazel (sore)

Breathing:

Secondary:
Butcher's Broom - decoction with honey (difficulty)
Coltsfoot - juice or syrup (shortness)

Other Possible:
Barberry (slows)

Bronchitis:

Primary:
Angelica (chronic)
Anise - oil mixed with wine
Black Cohosh (chronic)
Chickweed
Coltsfoot
Elder - berries
Elecampane
Fennel
Garlic - syrup
Green Tea
Horehound
Licorice
Lobelia
Marshmallow - boiled in wine or milk
Mullein
Pennyroyal
Pleurisy
Red Clover - infusion
Slippery Elm - drink - see page
Yerba Santa

Secondary:
Catnip
Cloves
Couch Grass
Damiana
Golden Seal
Kava Kava
Myrrh
Psyllium
Sage
Saw Palmetto (chronic, sedative)
St. John's Wort
Tea Tree

Other Possible:
Barberry (constriction)
Boneset
Elder - flowers
Horsetail
External:
Lavender – vapors

Bruises:

External:

Agrimony
Arnica (reduces)
Balm of Gilead - with lard or oil
Burdock
Caraway - poultice
Chickweed
Comfrey
Elder - leaves - ointment
Hops
Hyssop - leaves
Lady's Mantle
Lobelia
Marshmallow
Pennyroyal - green herb, bruised
Rosemary - bath
Shepherd's Purse - bruised herb
Solomon's Seal - poultice
St. John's Wort
Violet - leaves
White Willow - compress
Witch Hazel
Wormwood - poultice
Yarrow

Burns:

External:

Alfalfa
Aloe Vera
Balm of Gilead - simmered with oil
Barberry (reduce risk of infection)
Comfrey
Elder - flower water
Ginger (minor)
Gotu Kola
Horsetail - poultice
Hyssop - wash
Lavender – oil (very good)
Mullein
Raspberry Leaf - poultice with slippery elm
Slippery Elm - poultice - see page
St. John's Wort
White Oak
Witch Hazel

Secondary:

Astragalus

Bursitis:

Secondary:

Turmeric

Calming to Body:

Primary:

Boneset
Scullcap

Cancer:

Primary:
Astragalus
Burdock
Cat's Claw
Cayenne (lung)
Dandelion (tumors)
Echinacea
Frankincense (tumors)
Garlic
Ginger (nausea with chemotherapy)
Green Tea
Parsley (prevent cell multiplication)
Pau D'Arco
Saw Palmetto (prostate)
Violet - leaves, infusion (pain, throat, tongue tumors - dissolves & heals)

Secondary:
Agrimony (helps produce "B" cells)
Aloe Vera
Butcher's Broom (tumors)
Chaste Tree (fibroid tumors)
Cloves, stomach (protects against)
Gingko Biloba
Hawthorne (leukemia)
Licorice
Milk Thistle
Mistletoe
Red Clover (preventative)
Rosemary
St, John's Wort (especially breast)
Turmeric
Violet Flowers (tumors, dissolves & heals)

Other Possible:
Alfalfa (chemotherapy effects)
Chamomile (endometrial)
Cinnamon (liver & melanoma)
Gingko Biloba
Poke - root (breasts - be careful)
Schizandra (skin)
Yucca (anti-cancer & tumors)

External:
Aloe Vera (radiation exposure)
Elder - flower water (tumors)
Garlic (tumors)
Milk Thistle - decoction
Poke - root - bath
Red Clover (growths)
Solomon's Seal - poultice (tumors)
St. John's Wort (tumors)
Witch Hazel - poultice (tumors)

Candida:
See Yeast

Canker Sores:

External:
Burdock
Golden Seal - wash
Myrrh
Raspberry Leaf
Sage – wash

Carbuncles:

External:
Chickweed - poultice in muslin - one of the best

Cardiovascular Diseases:

Primary:
Gotu Kola (congestive heart failure)
Hawthorne (strengthens heart & increases flow of blood & oxygen, restores heart muscle)
Hops
Mistletoe
Scullcap

Secondary:
Astragalus
Cramp Bark
Garlic (preventative)
Hops

Carpal Tunnel Syndrome:

Primary:
Devil's Claw

Secondary:
Butcher's Broom
St. John's Wort
Turmeric

Other Possible:
Corn Silk

External:
Arnica

Cataracts:

See also Eyes

Primary:
Bilberry - fruit

Secondary:
Turmeric (prevents, over many years)

Celiac Disease:

Secondary:
Licorice

Chicken Pox:

Primary:
Yarrow

Secondary:
Catnip

Chronic Fatigue Syndrome:

Secondary:
Echinacea

Circulation:

Primary:
Bayberry
Blessed Thistle
Butcher's Broom (disorders, especially legs)
Cinnamon
Garlic
Ginger (stimulant)
Gingko Biloba (all, especially brain)
Gotu Kola
Hawthorne (disorders)
Horseradish
Rosemary
Scullcap
Valerian

Secondary:
Angelica (promotes to extremities)
Honeysuckle (increases blood flow to dermis)

Other Possible:
Chickweed (problems)
Hyssop (problems)
Pleurisy - with Angelica & sassafras (equalizes)

External:
Black Pepper (increases)
Cayenne
Elecampane (increases & produces red skin)
Honeysuckle - warm oil (restores to extremities numbed by cold)
Rosemary

Cirrhosis:

See also Liver

Primary:

Agrimony
Dandelion - leaf
Green Tea
Milk Thistle
Turmeric

Secondary:

Couch Grass - juice of roots, drink frequently

Cold Sores:

See Mouth

Colds:

Primary:

Angelica - hot tea
Anise
Astragalus
Blue Vervain
Boneset
Catnip
Cayenne
Chamomile
Echinacea
Elder - berries
Elder - flowers - hot tea at bedtime
Feverfew
Garlic
Ginger - tea
Golden Seal
Horehound
Ma Huang
Marshmallow
Myrrh
Pennyroyal - warm infusion
Peppermint – tea (slight)
Rosemary - tea
Sage - tea
Thyme - tea
Yarrow - tea with cayenne (severe)

Secondary:

Bayberry - hot tea
Burdock
Cat's Claw
Coltsfoot - decoction or tea
Hyssop
Pau D'Arco
Sarsaparilla - syrup
Saw Palmetto
Slippery Elm
Violet - leaves
White Willow

Other Possible:

Caraway - tea
Chickweed
Cinnamon
Comfrey
Eyebright
Lavender
Licorice
Sassafras (preventative)
Valerian (head)
Yerba Santa

External:

Balm of Gilead - ointment (shortens)
Eucalyptus - inhale steam
Tea Tree - oil, gargle with water

Colic:

Primary:

Angelica
Anise - star anise
Blue Cohosh
Catnip
Echinacea
Ginger
Peppermint
Rosemary - tea
Valerian

Secondary:

Anise - see recipe
Caraway
Chamomile
Elder - berries
Fennel
Parsley
Peppermint

(Colic, cont'd.)

Other Possible:
Centuary - decoction
Pennyroyal

Colitis:

Primary:
Chamomile
Ginger
Marshmallow - one of the best
Nettles
Slippery Elm
Yarrow

Secondary:
Agrimony
Cascara Sagrada
Psyllium

Colon Disorders:

Primary:
Alfalfa
Barley Grass
Golden Seal (inflammation)
Mullein - with milk (bleeding)
Nettles (all)

Secondary:
Licorice (cleanses)
Rhubarb

Concentration:

Primary:
Gingko Biloba

Congestion:

Primary:
Coltsfoot
Hyssop

Secondary:
Bayberry - hot tea
Ma Huang

Other Possible:
Juniper

Congestive Heart Failure:

Secondary:
Elecampane (pain)

Conjunctivitis:

External:
Fennel – compress

Connective Tissue:

Primary:
Horsetail (heals & strengthens)

Secondary:
Bilberry - fruit (strengthens & prevents degeneration)

Constipation:

Primary:

Alfalfa
Aloe Vera
Barberry (purgative)
Basil
Black Walnut
Boneset - cold drink
Cascara Sagrada
Damiana
Dandelion
Elder - berries (mild)
Elder - bark & leaves (strong purgative)
Fennel (gentle)
Ginger (cramping)
Golden Seal (habitual)
Mullein
Psyllium
Rhubarb
Senna

Secondary:

Black Pepper
Blue Vervain (painless)
Borage (mild)
Butcher's Broom
Chickweed - fresh decoction
Dong Quai
Elder - flower tea (gentle)
Fenugreek
Horehound (purgative, gentle)
Milk Thistle
Oregon Grape - with cascara sagrada
Slippery Elm (children)
Violet - flowers - syrup (slight)

Other Possible:

Allspice - water, as vehicle for other purgatives
Dong Quai
Pleurisy
Violet - leaves

External:

Slippery Elm (enema)

Convulsions:

See Anticonvulsant

Corns:

External:

Dandelion

Coughs:

See also Expectorant

Primary:

Agrimony
Angelica (facilitates other expectorants)
Anise (hard & dry coughs)
Balm of Gilead
Black Cohosh
Blue Vervain
Boneset
Chickweed - infusion
Coltsfoot - juice with marshmallow & horehound, or smoke leaves
Comfrey
Elecampane (expectorant)
Fennel - syrup with honey
Feverfew - with honey
Garlic - syrup
Horehound (chronic & smokers)
Horseradish - with honey & warm water
Hyssop (expectorant)
Licorice
Marshmallow - boiled in wine or milk
Mullein - boiled in wine or milk; smoke (hacking)
Myrrh
Nettles
Pennyroyal
Peppermint (nagging)
Pleurisy (spasmodic)
Sage
Slippery Elm - compound
St. John's Wort
Thyme - steam or oil
Violet - fresh flowers
Yerba Santa (nagging)

(Coughs, cont'd.)

Secondary:

Bayberry - hot tea
Couch Grass
Elder - berries
Fenugreek
Gingko Biloba (expectorant)
Parsley
Pau D'Arco
Red Clover
Sarsaparilla - syrup
Saw Palmetto
Solomon's Seal
Tea Tree (expectorant)

Other Possible:

Caraway - tea
Elder - leaves & flowers - tea
Ginger
Lavender - steam

External:

Anise - smoke & seeds
Horehound - lozenge

Crabs:

External:

Thyme – extract

Cramps – Menstrual:

Primary:

Black Cohosh
Blue Cohosh
Chamomile
Comfrey
Cramp Bark (all)
Dandelion - leaf
Dong Quai
False Unicorn
Pennyroyal (due to suppression)
Primrose
Raspberry Leaf
Rosemary
Scullcap
Valerian
Yarrow

Secondary:

Catnip
Cinnamon
Ginger
Lady's Slipper
Rosemary
St. John's Wort

Other Possible:

Angelica
Chickweed
Honeysuckle - leaves infused in oil
Sage
Turmeric

Crohn's Disease:

Primary:

St. John's Wort

Secondary:

Fennel
Licorice
Marshmallow
Milk Thistle
Peppermint
Psyllium
Slippery Elm

Croup:

Primary:

Thyme

Cuts:

External:
Barberry (kills bacteria)
Chamomile - cream
Comfrey
Eucalyptus - ointment
Hyssop – green herb bruised (quick heal)
Lavender (antibacterial)
Lobelia
Mullein
Myrrh
Rosemary
Solomon's Seal
St. John's Wort
Tea Tree - oil (disinfects)
White Willow – compress
Witch Hazel
Yarrow

Cystitis:

Primary:
Buchu
Cranberry
Nettles

Secondary:
Burdock
Corn Silk (acute & chronic)
Juniper
Tea Tree

Other Possible:
Alfalfa
Couch Grass

External:
Tea Tree - oil

D.T.'s:
See also Alcoholism

Primary:
Hops
Lady's Slipper

Secondary:
Scullcap

Other Possible:
Chamomile

Dandruff:

External:
Burdock
Ginger - with olive oil
Rosemary - with olive oil
Tea Tree - oil
White Willow - infusion of bark & leaves

Decongestant:

External:
Eucalyptus

Delirium:

Primary:
Blue Vervain
Hops
Mistletoe

Deodorant:

External:
Myrrh
Thyme
White Willow - with borax

Dental Problems:
See Teeth, Gums

Depressant:

Other Possible:
Sculleap (central nervous system)
Juniper

Depression:

Primary:
Damiana
Feverfew
Gotu Kola
Lavender
Rosemary - tea (nervous)
Schizandra
Scullcap
St. John's Wort (nervous)

Secondary:
Blue Vervain
Kava Kava (anxiety related)

Other Possible:
Gingko Biloba
Licorice

Dermatitis:
See Skin

Detox:

Primary:
Alfalfa (especially liver)
Black Cohosh
Black Walnut - leaves
Bladderwrack
Burdock - one of the best
Centuary
Dandelion
Echinacea
Garlic
Golden Seal
Gotu Kola
Hops - juice
Oregon Grape Root (liver & blood)
Pau D'Arco
Raspberry Leaf
Red Clover - extract
Sage - tea
Sarsaparilla
Sassafras
Turmeric (liver)
Violet - leaves - one of the best

Secondary:
Agrimony
Blessed Thistle
Boneset
Cat's Claw (intestines)
Couch Grass
Elder - leaves & flowers
Elecampane
Nettles
Pennyroyal
Queen of the Meadow
Yucca

Other Possible:
Chickweed
Cloves
Corn Silk
False Unicorn
Licorice
Milk Thistle
Poke - root
Violet - flowers
Yerba Santa

Diabetes:

Primary:
Bilberry - leaves - tea
Blue Cohosh
Burdock
Fenugreek
Golden Seal (increases effectiveness of insulin)
Green Tea

Secondary:
Agrimony (lowers sugar)
Alfalfa - with manganese
Aloe Vera
Astragalus
Cat's Claw
Cayenne
Cinnamon
Garlic
Ginkgo Biloba (retinopathy)
Milk Thistle (insulin resistance)
Nettles (preventative)
Pau D'Arco (prevent glucose in urine)

External:
Cayenne - cream (nerve damage)

Diaper Rash:

External:
Chamomile

Diarrhea:

Primary:
Agrimony
Bilberry - fruit - syrup with slippery elm
Black Cohosh (children's)
Cinnamon
Comfrey
Ginger
Mullein - with milk
Nettles
Peppermint
Queen of the Meadow (especially children)
Raspberry Leaf (children's)
Rhubarb
Rose Hips - tea
Slippery Elm
St. John's Wort
White Willow (chronic)
Witch Hazel - bark tea (acute but not chronic)
Yarrow

Secondary:
Barberry
Catnip
Garlic
Lady's Mantle (violent purging, halts)
Passion Flower
Pleurisy
Psyllium
White Oak
Yerba Santa

Other Possible:
Bayberry
Black Pepper
Coltsfoot
Dragon's Blood
Elder - berries
Guarana (mild)
Hawthorne
Oregon Grape (bacterial)
Pennyroyal

Digestion:

Primary:

Alfalfa (disorders)
Agrimony (promotes)
Anise (languid)
Astragalus
Black Pepper (aids with meals)
Catnip
Cayenne
Chamomile
Cinnamon
Cloves
Damiana
Dandelion
Ginger
Golden Seal
Horseradish - with orange peel, nutmeg & wine (languid)
Nutmeg (promotes)
Oregon Grape (improves)
Parsley
Pau D'Arco
Peppermint (enhances by increasing stomach acidity)
Sage - tea
White Willow

Secondary:

Barberry (regulates)
Basil
Buchu (disorders)
Caraway (disorders)
Centuary
Chickweed (helps system)
Devil's Claw (soothes)
Fennel (soothes)
Juniper (problems)
Rosemary
Slippery Elm (irritation)
Wormwood - see page (improves)
Yarrow

Other Possible:

Angelica (problems)
Hawthorne (problems)

Disinfectant:

External:

Eucalyptus
Garlic
Myrrh
Tea Tree - oil
Thyme

Diuretic:

Primary:
Alfalfa
Agrimony
Astragalus
Bilberry
Black Cohosh
Blue Cohosh
Buchu
Burdock
Butcher's Broom
Catnip
Chamomile
Corn Silk
Couch Grass - infusion
Cranberry
Damiana
Dandelion
Elder - berries
Elecampane
Fennel - tea (safe)
Garlic
Gotu Kola
Gravel Root
Hops
Horseradish
Horsetail
Juniper - oil
Kava Kava
Parsley
Queen of the Meadow - tea
Sarsaparilla
Saw Palmetto
Shepherd's Purse
Slippery Elm
St. John's Wort
Yarrow

(Diuretic, cont'd.)

Secondary:
Angelica (mild)
Balm of Gilead
Borage
Devil's Claw
Elder - leaves
False Unicorn
Hawthorne
Honeysuckle
Horehound
Marshmallow
Mullein
Passion Flower
Pennyroyal
Rose Hips
Rosemary
Thyme

Other Possible:
Anise - star anise
Chickweed
Elder - bark
Guarana
Ma Huang
Pleurisy
Sassafras

Diverticulitis:

Primary:
Chamomile

Dizziness:

Primary:
Gingko Biloba

Secondary:
Peppermint
Rosemary
Schizandra

Other Possible:
Feverfew

Dog Bites:

Secondary:
Burdock

Douche:

Chamomile
Comfrey
Golden Seal (fungal infections)
Lady's Mantle (soothing)
Lavender
Marshmallow
Myrrh
Sage
Slippery Elm
Thyme (pain)
White Oak
Yarrow

Dropsy (Edema):

Primary:
Astragalus
Bilberry - fruit, bruised with roots & steeped in gin
Butcher's Broom
Gravel Root
Horseradish
Parsley

Secondary:
Corn Silk
Hawthorne
Horsetail
Queen of the Meadow
Shepherd's Purse

Other Possible:
Alfalfa (relieves)
Centuary
Elder - leaves
Elecampane
Juniper - spirits (cardiac, stimulating diuretic)

Drug Withdrawal:

See also D.T.'s

Secondary:
Scullcap

Dysentery:

Primary:
Comfrey
Peppermint
Solomon's Seal - infusion (chronic)
St. John's Wort
White Willow
Witch Hazel

Secondary:
Bilberry - fruit, syrup
Frankincense
Ginger
Shepherd's Purse
Slippery Elm

Other Possible:
Mullein
Pleurisy
Poke - root
Psyllium
Rhubarb

E. Coli:

Primary:

Agrimony
Bilberry

Other Possible:

Oregon Grape Root

External:

Tea Tree – oil

Ear Infection:

External:

Echinacea - with goldenseal
Garlic - oil
Green Tea

Ear Pain:

Primary:

Gingko Biloba (ringing)
Hops

External:

Chamomile
Garlic - oil
Ginger - warm oil
Mullein - oil
Shepherd's Purse - juice drops

Eczema:

Primary:

Nettles
Primrose (especially infantile)

Secondary:

Black Walnut
Burdock
Dandelion
Sarsaparilla

Other Possible:

Gingko Biloba
Pleurisy
Red Clover

External:

Aloe Vera
Black Walnut
Burdock - see page
Chamomile
Chickweed
Dandelion
Echinacea
Elder - berries
Golden Seal
Green Tea
Lavender
Marshmallow
Oregon Grape
Red Clover
Rosemary - bath
Sarsaparilla
Witch Hazel

Edema:

See Dropsy

Emmenagogue:

Primary:
Angelica - tea
Black Cohosh
Blessed Thistle
Blue Cohosh
Catnip - cold juice
Fennel
Feverfew
Myrrh - one of the best
Pennyroyal

Secondary:
Blue Vervain
Boneset
Thyme

Other Possible:
Anise
Centuary
Henna - fruit
Horsetail - strong decoction
Yarrow

Emotional Upset:

Primary:
Passion Flower (extreme)
St. John's Wort

Emphysema:
See also Lungs

Secondary:
Damiana

Other Possible:
Licorice

Endometriosis:

Primary:
Green Tea

Secondary:
Alfalfa
Gravel Root
Turmeric

Epilepsy:

Primary:
Blue Cohosh
Blue Vervain
Lavender - see page
Lobelia
Mistletoe
Scullcap
Thyme
Valerian

Secondary:
Passion Flower

Other Possible:
Anise
Elder - bark & berries
Hyssop
Violet - flowers, syrup

Episiotomy:

Secondary:
Gotu Kola (heals)

Erectile Dysfunction:

Secondary:
Sarsaparilla

Eruptions:

External:
Honeysuckle – bark, lotion

Estrogen:

Primary:
Chaste Tree (replacement therapy)

Secondary:
Primrose (promotes)
Sage (deficiency)

Exhaustion:

Primary:
Guarana

Secondary:
Sarsaparilla (increases energy)

Expectorant:
See also coughs

Primary:
Angelica (facilitates other expectorants)
Elecampane
Hyssop

Secondary:
Gingko Biloba
Tea Tree

Eyes:

Primary:
Bilberry - fruit (general & eyestrain)
Eyebright (disease & weakness)

Secondary:
Black Cohosh (blurred vision)
Dong Quai (prevents retinal swelling)
Schizandra (vision)
Violet Flowers - syrup (inflammation)

Other Possible:
Chamomile
Cloves
Dandelion
Gingko Biloba

External:
Anise - wash (soothing)
Angelica - drops & poultice (problems)
Bayberry
Chickweed - juice (hot & red)
Elder - leaves, ointment (inflammation)
Elder - flowers, cold tea (inflammation)
Eyebright - see page (inflammation, pain, allergies, itchy, strain, all)
Fennel - water (tired & sore)
Golden Seal - wash (sore)
Horsetail (eyelid swelling)
Marshmallow - wash
Myrrh (infections)
Pennyroyal - green herb bruised
Sassafras - wash in rosewater - see page
Witch Hazel - wash (eyelid inflammation)

Faintness:

Primary:
Lavender - oil

External:
Pennyroyal - applied to nostrils with vinegar

Fatigue:

Primary:
Astragalus
Gotu Kola
Green Tea (mental)
Guarana
Schizandra
Valerian

Secondary:
Licorice
Scullcap

External:
Lavender – bath

Feet:

External:
Arnica - hot footbath (tender)
Sage - bath (tired)
Witch Hazel (tired)

Fever:

Primary:
Agrimony
Bayberry (reduces)
Blessed Thistle - warm infusion
Blue Vervain
Boneset - one of the best (all)
Catnip
Centuary (intermittent)
Chamomile
Coltsfoot
Elder - berries, wine (promotes perspiration)
Fenugreek
Feverfew
Gotu Kola
Lobelia
Queen of the Meadow - infusion of fresh tops
Sage - tea
Sarsaparilla
Thyme - tea
White Oak
White Willow
Yarrow - tea with cayenne (severe)

Secondary:
Angelica
Black Pepper
Borage
Fennel
Frankincense
Ginger
Hyssop
Parsley
Peppermint
Pleurisy - with angelica & sassafras

Other Possible:
Balm of Gilead
Barberry (intermittent)
Bilberry - fruit
Black Cohosh
Dandelion
Guarana (reduces)
Hops
Horehound
Horsetail (cools)
Juniper
Rhubarb
Shepherd's Purse
Violet - leaves, drink

External:
Catnip - one of the best (enema)
Violet - leaves, plaster (cools)

Fibromyalgia:

Other Possible:
Licorice

Fits:

Primary:
Cramp Bark

Flea Repellant:

External:
Eucalyptus - oil (kills)
Fennel
Pennyroyal
Wormwood - stuffed in beds of cats & dogs

Flu:

Primary:
Anise
Astragalus
Blue Vervain
Boneset - one of the best
Catnip
Echinacea
Elder - berries, wine, hot at night (promotes perspiration)
Elder - flowers - strong infusion with peppermint at bedtime
Garlic
Golden Seal
Green Tea
Myrrh - one of the best (stomach)
Thyme
Yarrow

(Flu, cont'd.)

Secondary:
Bayberry
Black Pepper
Burdock
Ginger - tea
Ma Huang (with low blood pressure due to flu)
Mullein
Queen of the Meadow
Slippery Elm

External:
Balm of Gilead - ointment (shortens)
Eucalyptus - inhale steam

Food Poisoning:

Primary:
Green Tea

Secondary:
Cayenne
Cloves
Fennel
Peppermint
Slippery Elm

Fractures:

External:
Arnica

Frostbite:

External:
Aloe Vera

Fungal Infections:
See Anti-fungal

Gallbladder:

Primary:
Burdock (restores function)
Dandelion
Oregon Grape (stimulative)
Turmeric (disease)

Secondary:
Horsetail (problems)

Other Possible:
Blue Vervain
Milk Thistle (disease)

Gallstones:

Primary:
Cascara Sagrada
Dandelion - root
Turmeric
White Oak

Secondary:
Barberry
Juniper
Parsley
Peppermint

Other Possible:
Milk Thistle

Gangrene:

Other Possible:
Henna

External:
Arrowroot
Comfrey - hot poultice (wounds)
Garlic (preventative)
Henna
Lady's Mantle
Slippery Elm - poultice

Gas:

Primary:
Angelica (quick & safe for children)
Anise - with Caraway
Basil
Black Pepper
Caraway
Catnip
Cayenne (relieves)
Chamomile
Cinnamon
Cloves
Fennel - tea (especially in children) - one of the
best & safest
Feverfew
Ginger
Golden Seal
Juniper - oil (cramps)
Parsley
Peppermint - spirit in hot water (pain)
Pleurisy
Sage
Slippery Elm
Thyme - tea
Valerian

Secondary:
Garlic
Hops
Horehound
Hyssop
Lavender
Nutmeg
Yarrow

Other Possible:
Anise - star anise
Horehound
Myrrh
Queen of the Meadow

Gastritis:

Primary:
Ginger (alcoholic)
Marshmallow
St. John's Wort

Secondary:
Cat's Claw
Mullein

Germicide:

Extract:
Cloves (strong)
Thyme

Gingivitis:

External:
Cinnamon
Myrrh

Glandular Swelling:

Primary:
Golden Seal
Mullein

Secondary:
Echinacea

Glaucoma:

Secondary:
Hawthorne

Other Possible:
Ginkgo Biloba

Gleet:

Primary:
Witch Hazel

External:
Dragon's Blood – douche

Goiter:

Primary:
Parsley
White Oak

Gonorrhea:

Primary:
Echinacea
Hops
Kava Kava
Sassafras

Secondary:
Corn Silk
Parsley

Other Possible:
Yerba Santa

External:
Frankincense
Golden Seal

Gout:

Primary:

Agrimony
Burdock - tea
Dandelion
Devil's Claw (pain)
Fenugreek
Gravel Root
Juniper
Red Clover
Sarsaparilla (pain)
Wormwood

Secondary:

Bilberry
Centuary
Fennel
Kava Kava
Nettles
Parsley
Pennyroyal
St. John's Wort - tea
Thyme

Other Possible:

Angelica - stem juice, dried
Blue Vervain
Comfrey
Couch Grass
Hyssop
Sassafras

External:

Angelica - compress
Burdock - poultice
Rosemary
Thyme

Gravel:

Primary:

Bilberry - fruit, bruised with roots & steeped in gin
Butcher's Broom - infusion
Corn Silk
Couch Grass (relieves)

Secondary:

Horsetail

Griping:

Primary:

Anise (diminishes)
Pennyroyal

Secondary:

Allspice - 2-3 drops oil on sugar

Gums:

Secondary:

Thyme

Other Possible:

Marshmallow

External:

Bayberry - wash (sore)
Buchu (inflammation)
Chamomile
Goldenseal (inflamed)
Myrrh (spongy & soft)
Sage - gargle (bleeding)
Witch Hazel (sore)

Hair:

Primary:

Horsetail (strengthens & eliminates oil)

Other Possible:

Yarrow

External:

Arnica - apply to scalp (growth)
Black Walnut (colors)
Burdock (loss)
Catnip (encourages growth)
Chamomile (brightens)
Comfrey (dry)
Ginger - tea (growth)
Lavender (greasy)
Marshmallow (dry)
Nettles, greasy - lotion (growth)
Sage - rinse (growth)

Halitosis:
See Bad Breath

Hands:

External:
Elder - flowers, ointment (chapped)

Hangover:
See also Alcoholism

Primary:
Cayenne
Ginger

Secondary:
Aloe Vera
Guarana

Hay Fever:

Primary:
Mullein
Yerba Santa

Secondary:
Ma Huang
Nettles

Other Possible:
Eyebright
Horehound

Headache:

Primary:
Blue Vervain
Chamomile
Damiana
Feverfew - one of the best (migraine)
Guarana (rheumatic, nervous & menstrual)
Lady's Slipper
Lavender - tea (nervous)
Rhubarb
Rosemary - oil & tea
Sage - infusion, strong (nervous)
Scullcap - one of the best (nervous)
St. John's Wort (fever & tension)
Thyme - tea
Valerian
White Willow

Secondary:
Black Cohosh
Cloves
Kava Kava
Passion Flower (nervous)
Pennyroyal
Peppermint - tea
Poke - root
Rose Hips
Schizandra
Violet - flowers, syrup

Other Possible:
Coltsfoot
Eyebright
Ginger
Gingko Biloba
Honeysuckle - distilled water (nervous)
Mistletoe
Yerba Santa

External:
Blue Vervain - poultice
Elder - flower water on temples
Eucalyptus - oil on temples (tension)
Lavender - oil
Peppermint - oil on forehead
Yerba Santa - compress

Heart:

See also Cardiovascular Disease

Primary:

Blessed Thistle (strengthens)
Cayenne
Cramp Bark (palpitation)
Garlic (prevent attack)
Gotu Kola
Hawthorne (increases flow of blood & oxygen, restores muscle)
Lavender (nervous palpitation)
Peppermint (trouble with palpitation)
Scullcap (strengthens)

Secondary:

Astragalus (normalizes & improves circulation
after attack)
Cinnamon (prevent attack)
Dong Quai (attack)
Gingko Biloba (disorders)
Rosemary - with wine (stimulant)
Slippery Elm - drink
Turmeric (attack, reduce tissue damage)
Valerian (palpitations)
Yarrow (nervous condition)

Other Possible:

Barberry (decreases rate)
Chamomile
Horsetail (strengthens)
Mistletoe (slows beat)
Psyllium (disease)
Yarrow (slows beat)

Heartburn:

Primary:

Goldenseal
Licorice

Secondary:

Devil's Claw (soothes)

Other:

Angelica
Centuary
Peppermint

Heat Stress:

Secondary:

Cayenne

Hemorrhaging:

Primary:

Comfrey - one of the best (all internal)
Lady's Mantle - decoction
Mistletoe
Mullein (lungs)
Sage - tea (lungs & stomach)
Shepherd's Purse (all, especially kidneys & uterus)
Slippery Elm (all, especially lungs)
St. John's Wort - with knotgrass (spitting blood)
Witch Hazel (stomach)
Yarrow (all)

Secondary:

Cinnamon - with chalk (uterine)
White Oak (from mouth)

Other Possible:

Bayberry (all kinds)
Horsetail (spitting blood)
Rhubarb

External:

Bayberry (uterine)

Hemorrhoids:

Primary:
Butcher's Broom
Chamomile
Mullein - boiled in milk
Nettles - tea
Psyllium
Rhubarb
St. John's Wort
White Oak
Yerba Santa

Secondary:
Horsetail
Psyllium
Shepherd's Purse
Yarrow

Other Possible:
Alfalfa

External:
Aloe Vera
Bayberry
Burdock
Butcher's Broom (itching, burning & pain)
Chamomile
Comfrey
Echinacea - enema
Elder - flower, with honeysuckle in water or milk
Gingko Biloba
Golden Seal - enema
Mullein - poultice
Myrrh
Poke - root
Solomon's Seal - wash
Witch Hazel

Hepatitis:

Primary:
Dandelion
Gotu Kola
Milk Thistle

Secondary:
Licorice

Other Possible:
Red Clover

Hernia:

Secondary:
Fennel (heals)

Herpes:

Primary:
Black Walnut

Secondary:
Cat's Claw
Echinacea - extract
St. John's Wort

Other Possible:
Licorice

External:
Black Walnut
Cayenne - cream
Green Tea
Tea Tree – oil

Hiccups:

Primary:
- Fennel - tea
- Scullcap (severe)

Secondary:
- Honeysuckle

Other Possible:
- Anise
- Valerian

High Blood Pressure:

Primary:
- Black Cohosh
- Cayenne
- Garlic
- Golden Seal
- Gotu Kola
- Green Tea
- Hawthorne (reduces)
- Primrose

Secondary:
- Angelica
- Astragalus
- Bilberry
- Dandelion
- Devil's Claw
- Dong Quai
- Hyssop (regulates)
- Mistletoe
- Parsley
- Passion Flower
- Rosemary
- Schizandra
- Turmeric
- Valerian

Other Possible:
- Alfalfa
- Hawthorne
- Yarrow

High Blood Sugar:

Primary:
- Pau D'Arco

Secondary:
- Burdock
- Devil's Claw
- Nettles

Other Possible:
- Fenugreek
- Juniper (regulates)

High Cholesterol:

Primary:
- Black Cohosh
- Garlic
- Green Tea
- Hawthorne
- Thyme
- Turmeric

Secondary:
- Dandelion
- Ginger
- Milk Thistle
- Psyllium
- Primrose
- Rosemary
- Schizandra

Other Possible:
- Alfalfa

HIV:
See also AIDS

Primary:
Red Clover

Secondary:
Aloe Vera
Cat's Claw
Cinnamon
Licorice
Raspberry Leaf
Saw Palmetto (weight loss)
Turmeric

Other Possible:
St. John's Wort

Hives:

External:
Chamomile
Nettles (especially shellfish)
Sarsaparilla

Hoarseness:

Primary:
Chickweed - infusion
Garlic - syrup
Licorice - with rosewater

Secondary:
Mullein
Violet - flowers

Other Possible:
Yerba Santa

External:
Horehound - lozenge
Lavender – gargle

Hormonal Balance:

Primary:
Saw Palmetto (regulates)

Secondary:
Sarsaparilla (regulates)

Other Possible:
Alfalfa

Hot Flashes:

Primary:
Black Cohosh
Dong Quai - one of the best
Primrose
Raspberry Leaf

Secondary:
Damiana
Ginger
Sage

Hydrophobia:

Primary:
Scullcap

Secondary:
Chickweed - with Elecampane

Hyperactivity:

Primary:
Hops
Passion Flower
Scullcap

Other Possible:
Primrose

Hypochondria:

Primary:
Damiana
Valerian

Secondary:
Dandelion
Lady's Slipper

Hypoglycemia:

Primary:
Golden Seal

Secondary:
Bilberry - leaves & root
Licorice

Hysteria:

Primary:
Cramp Bark
Feverfew
Hops
Lady's Slipper
Mistletoe
Passion Flower
Scullcap
St. John's Wort
Valerian

Secondary:
Blue Cohosh
Pennyroyal - water

Other Possible:
Black Cohosh
Caraway
Cranberry
Garlic
Peppermint – infusion

Immune System:

Primary:
Alfalfa (stimulates)
Astragalus (depression, stimulates)
Burdock (stimulates)
Cat's Claw
Echinacea
Golden Seal

Other Possible:
Bayberry - hot tea
Hawthorne (boosts)
Horehound (boosts)
Milk Thistle (weakened)

Impotency:

Primary:
Damiana
False Unicorn
Gingko Biloba (increases blood supply)
Sarsaparilla
Schizandra

Indigestion:

Primary:

Angelica
Cayenne
Chamomile
Cinnamon
Cloves
Fennel
Feverfew
Garlic
Ginger
Licorice
Marshmallow
Parsley
Peppermint
Turmeric
Valerian (nervous)

Secondary:

Anise
Boneset - infusion
Devil's Claw
Hops
Juniper - oil
Pleurisy - rarely used
Rosemary
Slippery Elm

Other Possible:

Angelica (heartburn)
Centuary
Elecampane
Hyssop
Oregon Grape
Peppermint
Primrose
Sage
Yarrow

Infantile Catarrh:

Other Possible:

Anise
Garlic

Infection:

Primary:

Cat's Claw
Cranberry (urinary & chronic kidney)
Echinacea (all)
Garlic (all, especially yeast)
Golden Seal
Gotu Kola (urinary)
Pau D'Arco (parasitic)
Rose Hips (all)
Yarrow (viral)

Secondary:

Alfalfa (urinary & bladder)
Angelica (urinary organ disease)
Astragalus (frequently occurring)
Cinnamon (yeast & fungal)
Gravel Root (kidney)
Kava Kava (urinary tract)
St. Johns' Wort (viral)

Other Possible:

Anise
Guarana (urinary)

External:

Balm of Gilead (wounds)
Nettles (yeast)
Pau D'Arco (fungal)

Infertility:

Primary:

Damiana
False Unicorn

Secondary:

Astragalus (male)
Black Cohosh (male)
Dong Quai (male)

Other Possible:

Sarsaparilla

Inflammation:

See Anti-inflammatory

Influenza:

See Flu

Insects:

External:

Aloe Vera (bites)
Anise - oil, with sassafras & carbolic oils
Arrowroot (bites & stings)
Basil (flies, repels)
Blessed Thistle (bites)
Burdock (bites)
Chamomile (repels)
Cloves (repels)
Comfrey (bites & stings, heals)
Elecampane - burn the herb (repels)
Eucalyptus - oil (bites, repels fleas, kills dust mites)
Fennel (repels flies)
Feverfew - tincture (bites)
Garlic (bites & mosquito larvae in ponds)
Juniper - oil mixed with lard (flies on wounds in animals)
Lavender (stings)
Lobelia (bites)
Parsley - poultice (stings)
Pennyroyal (repels fleas, flies, gnats, mosquitoes & ticks)
Peppermint (repels ants & aphids)
Sassafras - oil (repels fleas & moths)
Tea Tree - oil (bites)
White Oak (bee stings)
Witch Hazel (bites)
Wormwood (repellant on clothes, pantry, etc.)

Insomnia:

Primary:

Catnip
Chamomile
Garlic
Hops - tea (overwrought brain)
Kava Kava
Lady's Slipper
Lavender
Mullein
Passion Flower
Scullcap
Slippery Elm - drink (see recipe)
St. John's Wort (promotes deep sleep)
Valerian (esp. chronic)

Secondary:

Dong Quai
Schizandra
Violet - flowers, syrup

Other Possible:

Anise - a few drops in hot milk
Dandelion
Hawthorne
Lobelia
Peppermint

External:

Lady's Mantle - pillow
Lavender – pillow

Insulin:

Primary:

Bilberry - leaves (controls levels)
Bilberry - roots (controls levels)

Intestinal Worms:
See Worms

Intestines:

Primary:
Raspberry Leaf (spasms)

Secondary:
Cat's Claw (detox, replenish friendly bacteria)
Marshmallow
Parsley

Other Possible:
Comfrey
Corn silk (small intestines, aids)
Garlic

Irritable Bowel Syndrome:
See also Colon Disorders

Primary:
Slippery Elm
Valerian (spasms)

Secondary:
Chamomile
Comfrey
Dandelion - 15 days minimum
Licorice
Milk Thistle
Peppermint (blocks contractions)
Psyllium
Rosemary (cramps, bloating, gas)

Other Possible:
Milk Thistle

External:
St. John's Wort – enema

Irritability:

Primary:
Evening Primrose
Lady's Slipper (nervous)
Scullcap
Valerian

Irritation:

Primary:
Aloe Vera (stomach)
Saw Palmetto (sex organs, especially male)

External:
Arnica – ointment, see recipe (nasal passage)
Belladonna (skin)
Chickweed
Saw Palmetto (sex organs)

Itching:

External:
Blessed Thistle
Hops
Parsley
Sage
Witch Hazel

Jaundice:

Primary:
Agrimony - tea with honey
Barberry (all cases)
Borage
Butcher's Broom - infusion
Chamomile
Dandelion
Hops
Milk Thistle
Oregon Grape
Parsley
St. John's Wort
Turmeric

(Jaundice, cont'd.)

Secondary:
Couch Grass - juice of roots, drink frequently
Fennel
Wormwood (promotes bile)

Other Possible:
Bayberry - hot tea
Blessed Thistle
Centuary
Henna
Pennyroyal
Violet – flowers, syrup & leaves

Joints and Tissue:

Primary:
Alfalfa

External:
Witch Hazel (sore)

Kidney:

Primary:
Agrimony
Buchu (controls problems)
Burdock (all)
Butchers Broom (inflammation & tonic)
Corn Silk (inflammation)
Couch Grass (disease & inflammation)
Cranberry (chronic infections)
Damiana (clears)
Dandelion
Horsetail (especially stones)
Juniper - oil (diseases)
Parsley
Queen of the Meadow - one of the best (infection)
Raspberry Leaf
Sage - tea
White Oak
Yarrow

Secondary:
Astragalus (normalizes)
Balm of Gilead - tincture (complaints)
Borage (promotes activity)
Dong Quai (chronic inflammation)
Gingko Biloba (disorders)
Gravel Root (infection)
Hawthorne (troubles)
Kava Kava (pain)
Marshmallow
Passion Flower (complaints)
Red Clover
Shepherds Purse - with couch grass (complaints)

Other Possible:
Blessed Thistle
Centuary
Chamomile
Chickweed
False Unicorn (diseases)
Horseradish
Licorice (ailments)
Milk Thistle (protects)

Kidney Stones:

Primary:
Agrimony
Buchu
Gotu Kola
Parsley - tea (one of the best)

Secondary:
Aloe Vera
Gravel Root

Other Possible:
Barberry (preventative)
Chamomile

Labor:

Primary:
Black Cohosh (induces)
Blue Cohosh (induces)
Pennyroyal (facilitate, dangerous)
Raspberry Leaf (induces)

Secondary:
Gravel Root (pain)
Raspberry Leaf (pain)
Thyme (induces)

Other Possible:
Anise (facilitates)
Centuary (pain)

Laryngitis:

Primary:
Frankincense
Licorice
Lobelia
Marshmallow
Yerba Santa

Secondary:
Coltsfoot
Couch Grass
Tea Tree

Laxative:

See Constipation

Leg Cramps:

Primary:
Gingko Biloba (due to circulation)

Secondary:
Gotu Kola (swelling & pain)

Leprosy:

Primary:
Frankincense
Garlic

Secondary:
Henna

Other Possible:
Gotu Kola

External:
Sarsaparilla

Lethargy:

Primary:
Damiana

Leukemia:

Primary:
Pau D'Arco

Secondary:
Cascara Sagrada
Gravel Root
Hawthorne (accelerates death of cancer cells)

Other Possible:
Yarrow

Leucorrhoea:

Primary:
Blue Cohosh
Kava Kava

Secondary:
Black Cohosh

Other Possible:
Guarana (mild)
Juniper
Poke - root, tincture

External:
Bayberry
Poke - root, lotion

Lice:
See also Insects

External:
Angelica (itching)
Hyssop - oil
Lavender
Tea Tree - oil
Thyme – extract

Lips:

External:
Arnica (chapped)

Liver:
See also Cirrhosis

Primary:
Agrimony (all)
Alfalfa (detox)
Barberry (derangement)
Blessed Thistle
Burdock (restores, heals, protects)
Cascara Sagrada
Comfrey (ulcers)
Dandelion (disorders)
Garlic
Golden Seal
Gotu Kola (especially alcoholic, function)
Hops (sluggish)
Milk Thistle (all, heals, protects, stimulates new cell production)
Milk Thistle (obstructions, removes)
Oregon Grape (cleanses, sluggish, detox)
Parsley
Raspberry Leaf
Rhubarb
Rosemary (toxicity)
Sage (bilious)
Schizandra
Thyme (disease)
Turmeric (protects, cirrhosis, detox)

Secondary:
Corn Silk (disorders)
Dong Quai
Evening Primrose
Fennel
Red Clover
St. John's Wort
Wormwood (disease)
Yarrow

Other Possible:
Bilberry - fruit
Blue Vervain
Centuary
False Unicorn
Lavender
Peppermint (disorders)
Poke - root (regulates)

Lock Jaw:

Primary:
Cramp Bark

Low Blood Pressure:

Primary:
Blue Cohosh

Secondary:
Hyssop (regulates)
Schizandra

External:
Rosemary

Low Blood Sugar:

Other Possible:
Juniper (regulates)

Lungs:

Primary:
Astragalus (weak)
Cayenne
Chickweed (mucous buildup)
Coltsfoot
Comfrey (bleeding)
Elecampane (chronic diseases)
Fenugreek
Honeysuckle - flowers, syrup
Horehound (troubles)
Marshmallow - boiled in wine or milk
Mullein (bleeding)
Parsley
Pleurisy (inflammation)
Red Clover
Sassafras (damage from smoking)
Slippery Elm - drink (bleeding)
Solomon's Seal (inflamed)

(Lungs, cont'd.)

Secondary:
Blessed Thistle
Raspberry Leaf - smoke (irritation)
Violet - dried flowers (all diseases)

Other Possible:
Garlic
Horseradish (infection)
Horsetail (strengthen)
Mullein - smoke (irritation)

External:
Angelica - fresh leaf poultice (diseases)

Lupus:

Primary:
Nettles

Secondary:
Astragalus
Chamomile
Feverfew
Hawthorne
Licorice
Pau D'Arco

Lyme disease:

Secondary:
Cat's Claw
Echinacea
Licorice

Lymphatic System:

Primary:
Echinacea
Golden Seal

Malaria:

Secondary:
Barberry

Mastitis:

Secondary:
Fenugreek (promotes milk, eases pain)

External:
Marshmallow

Measles:

Primary:
Gotu Kola
Sage - tea
Yarrow - tea with cayenne

Secondary:
Burdock
Catnip

Melancholia:

Primary:
St. John's Wort

Secondary:
Thyme

Other Possible:
Cloves
Marshmallow

Memory:

Primary:
Blessed Thistle
Gingko Biloba - one of the best (loss of)
Sage

Secondary:
Blue Cohosh
Gotu Kola
Hawthorne (loss)
Lavender

Other Possible:
Cloves
Eyebright

Menopause:

See also Hot Flashes

Primary:
Black Cohosh
Chaste Tree (estrogen replacement therapy)
Dong Quai
Evening Primrose

Secondary:
Alfalfa (symptoms)
Cramp Bark
Damiana
Saw Palmetto (reduces hair growth)
Valerian

Other Possible:
Anise (symptoms)

Menstrual Cramps:

See Cramps

Menstrual Problems:

Primary:

Blue Cohosh (all disorders)
Blue Vervain
Cramp Bark (pain)
Dong Quai (irregularity)
False Unicorn (pain)
Guarana (headache)
Lady's Mantle - infusion (excessive)
Myrrh
Parsley (disorders)
Primrose (heavy bleeding)
Raspberry Leaf (excessive bleeding)
Shepherd's Purse (excessive)
White Willow (antiperiodic)
Yarrow

Secondary:

Chamomile (irregularities)
Cramp Bark (irregularity)
Gravel Root (pain)
Mistletoe (pain & spasms)
Witch Hazel (excessive)

Other Possible:

Rosemary (antiperiodic)
Sculleap (antiperiodic)

Mental Disorders:

Primary:

Catnip
Gotu Kola

Secondary:

Wormwood (restorative)

Metabolism:

Primary:

Astragalus (increases)
Cayenne

Other Possible:

Sarsaparilla (stimulates)

Migraine:

Primary:

Dong Quai (PMS induced)
Feverfew - one of the best
Henna
Mullein - tincture
Scullcap

Other Possible:

Blue Vervain
Cayenne
Mistletoe
Nettles
Peppermint
Wormwood

External:

Rosemary - oil rubbed on temples

Miscarriage:

Secondary:

Catnip (preventative)

Other Possible:

Cramp Bark (preventative)

Mold:

External:

Garlic (inhibits)

Mono:

Other Possible:
Red Clover

Morning Sickness:

Primary:
Black Cohosh
Ginger
Golden Seal
Raspberry Leaf - with peppermint

Secondary:
Catnip
Chamomile

Morphine Overdose:

Other Possible:
Schizandra

Mosquitoes:

External:
Basil (repels)

Mother's Milk:

Primary:
Anise (promotes)
Blessed Thistle (produces)
Fennel (stimulates)

Secondary:
Basil
Bilberry - fruit (stops)
Blue Vervain (increases)
Fenugreek (mastitis, promotes milk, eases pain)
Parsley
Raspberry Leaf

Other Possible:
Borage (increases)
Caraway (stimulates)
Hope
Lavender
Myrrh
Nettles (increases)
Sage (suppresses)

Moths:

External:
Pennyroyal (repels)

Motion Sickness:

Primary:
Fennel
Ginger - one of the best
Peppermint - tea

Other Possible:
Pennyroyal - see recipe

Mouth:

Secondary:
Thyme

Other Possible:
Marshmallow

External:
Barberry - gargle (sores)
Bilberry - leaves & bark (ulceration)
Black Walnut - gargle (sores)
Borage - gargle (ulcers)
Cloves - wash
Golden Seal (sores)
Hyssop (cold sores)
Myrrh - wash (sores)
St. John's Wort
Tea Tree - oil (cold sores)
Thyme - wash
Witch Hazel (cold sores)

Mucous:

See Phlegm

Primary:

Anise (clears from air passages)
Chickweed (buildup in lungs)
Thyme (reduces)

Secondary:

Corn Silk (in urine)
Oregon Grape (chronic complaints)
Shepherd's Purse (in urine)
White Oak (discharge)

Mucous Membranes:

Primary:

Golden Seal (inflamed)
Marshmallow (inflamed)

Secondary:

Bayberry (all conditions)
Ma Huang (swelling)

Other Possible:

Buchu (inflammation)

Muscle Cramps:

Primary:

Chamomile
Hops
Scullcap
Valerian

Secondary:

Kava Kava

Other Possible:

Horsetail
St. John's Wort

Muscle Relaxant:

Primary:

Feverfew
Red Clover
Scullcap
Valerian

Secondary:

Burdock
Cramp Bark
St. John's Wort

Other Possible:

Peppermint
Sassafras

Muscles – Sore:

External:

Arnica
Cayenne
Eucalyptus - ointment
Sage - bath
Witch Hazel

Muscle Spasms:

Primary:

Scullcap

Secondary:

Black Cohosh
Chamomile (preventative)
Cranberry (cramps & spasms)
Lavender

Muscle Strain:

Secondary:
Fennel

Muscular Dystrophy:

Secondary:
Gingko Biloba (prevent relapse)

Muscular Tissue:

Secondary:
Golden Seal
Saw Palmetto (building)

Nails:

Primary:
Borage (healthy)
Horsetail (strengthen)
Raspberry Leaf (healthy)

Other Possible:
Henna (brittle)

External:
Tea Tree - oil (infection)

Nasal Problems:

Other Possible:
Eyebright (running)
Sage

External:
Balm of Gilead - salve

Nausea:

Primary:
Basil - infusion
Cayenne
Cinnamon
Cloves - powder or infusion
Ginger (all, especially after surgery or chemotherapy)
Golden Seal
Peppermint - oil

Secondary:
Alfalfa
Anise
Black Pepper
Caraway
Nutmeg
St. John's Wort

Other Possible:
Pennyroyal

Nerves:

Primary:
Blue Vervain (complaints, preventative)
Borage (frazzled)
Catnip
Chamomile
Cramp Bark
Fennel - tea
Feverfew
Gotu Kola
Gravel Root
Hops
Kava Kava
Lady's Slipper
Lavender
Ma Huang (stimulant resembling adrenaline)
Mistletoe
Passion Flower
Rosemary
Scullcap
St. John's Wort
Valerian

(Nerves, cont'd.)

Secondary:
Basil
Black Cohosh (quietens & strengthens)
Frankincense
Guarana
Parsley
Thyme
Wormwood (tonic)

Other Possible:
Cranberry
Primrose

Nervous Disorders:

Primary:
Blue Cohosh
Chamomile
Guarana (headache)
Hops
Lady's Slipper (headaches)
Lavender - oil (palpitations)
Sage - tea (disease)
Scullcap (all, especially weakness & excitement)
Valerian (over-strain)

Secondary:
Pennyroyal - water
Peppermint - infusion

Other Possible:
Sarsaparilla (system disorders)

Night Blindness (Ophthalmia):

Primary:
Bilberry - fruit
Eyebright

External:
Chickweed - ointment
Eyebright

Nightmares:

Primary:
Catnip

Other Possible:
Turmeric

Night Sweats:

Secondary:
Sage

Nosebleed:

Primary:
Alfalfa (clots blood)

Secondary:
White Oak

External:
Shepherd's Purse - juice on cotton

Nursing:

Other Possible:
Alfalfa

Nutritive:

Primary:
Agar Agar - jelly (protein, for sick & infirm)
Alfalfa
Arrowroot (easy & pleasant, infant & invalid)
Barley Grass
Slippery Elm

Other Possible:
Licorice

Obesity:

Primary:
Bladderwrack
Chickweed - old wives remedy
Fennel - broth
Green Tea
Parsley

Secondary:
Cayenne - eat at breakfast (reduces appetite all
day & burns fat)
Cinnamon (metabolizes fat)
Dandelion
Nettles - seeds
Turmeric

Other Possible:
Anise (fat breakdown)
Butchers Broom
Corn silk
Hawthorne
Hyssop
Juniper

Osteoporosis:
See also Arthritis

Primary:
Yucca

Secondary:
Alfalfa
Dandelion
Hawthorne
White Willow

Other Possible:
Horsetail

Oxygen:

Primary:
Gingko Biloba (brain)

Pain:

Primary:
Catnip
Chamomile (especially back)
Comfrey
Devil's Claw
Dong Quai (ovarian cyst)
Ginger (stomach)
Hops
Lady's Slipper
Mullein
Nettles
Passion Flower (nerve pain)
Sage - tea (joint)
Scullcap (muscular)
St. John's Wort
Valerian
White Willow
Witch Hazel
Yucca (arthritis & rheumatism)

(Pain, cont'd.)

Secondary:
Black Cohosh
Chaste Tree (limbs)
Ginger
Golden Seal
Kava Kava (kidney & urinary)
Pau D'Arco
Slippery Elm (after vomiting)
Solomon's Seal (internal)
Thyme (hips)
Turmeric (shoulder)

Other Possible:
Lobelia
Primrose
Yucca (all)

External:
Arnica - one of the best
Belladonna
Cayenne
Chamomile (joint pain)
Comfrey
Elder - flowers
Eucalyptus
Hops - with chamomile
Lavender - hot in bags
Marshmallow
Myrrh
Peppermint (strains & sprains)
Rosemary - bath
Slippery Elm - poultice, see recipe
Thyme (aches)
Yarrow
Yerba Santa - poultice

Palsy:

Other Possible:
Chickweed

Pancreas:

Primary:
Golden Seal

Other Possible:
Barley Grass

Panic:

Primary:
Valerian (especially night attacks)

Paralysis:

Secondary:
Chaste Tree
Thyme

Other Possible:
Black Pepper
Mistletoe

External:
Black Pepper (tongue)

Parasites:

Primary:
Agrimony
Cloves
Garlic
Pau D'Arco (also River Blindness &
Chagas
Disease)

Secondary:
Bladderwrack
Cascara Sagrada
Ginger - see page
Thyme - oil (scabies)

External:
Black Walnut
Eucalyptus
Thyme - oil (scabies)

Parkinson's Disease:

Secondary:
Damiana
Gingko Biloba
Milk Thistle

Pelvic Inflammatory Disease:

Secondary:
Gravel Root

Periodontal Disease:

See also Teeth, Gums & Bleeding Gums

External:
Golden Seal - wash
Green Tea
Myrrh
Sage - gargle (bleeding gums)
Turmeric
Witch Hazel - gargle, mouthwash

Perspiration, Excessive:

Primary:
Black Walnut
Sage - tea

Secondary:
Schizandra

External:
Chamomile (odor)

Perspiration, Produces:

Primary:
Astragalus
Bayberry
Blessed Thistle
Blue Vervain
Boneset - warm infusion
Burdock
Cayenne
Elder - leaves, berry wine, flower tea
Garlic
Ginger
Lobelia
Pennyroyal - warm infusion
Rosemary
Sarsaparilla (profuse)
Sassafras
Yarrow - tea

Secondary:
Angelica
Elecampane
Honeysuckle (profuse)
Horehound
Hyssop
Pleurisy - warm infusion every hour
Queen of the Meadow - fresh tops, infusion
Thyme - tea

Other Possible:
Buchu
Butchers Broom
Centuary
Chamomile
Peppermint

Phlebitis:

Secondary:
Gingko Biloba
Gotu Kola

External:
Witch Hazel

Phlegm:
See also Mucous

Primary:
Angelica (buildup)
Boneset (loosens)
Borage (clears)
Coltsfoot (loosens)
Horehound - syrup (chest)
Licorice (increases fluidity)
Pennyroyal - with honey (clears)
Thyme

Secondary;
Butchers Broom
Yerba Santa

Other Possible:
Comfrey (loosens)
Lobelia

Piles:

Primary:
Witch Hazel - tea, one of the best (bleeding)

Other Possible:
Elder - berries

External:
Chickweed - ointment
Elder - leaves, boiled with linseed oil
Solomon's Seal - wash
Tea Tree
White Oak - ointment
Witch Hazel

Pimples:
See also Acne, Skin

External:
Agrimony
Senna
White Willow

Pituitary Gland:

Secondary:
Alfalfa (promotes function)

Placenta:

Other Possible:
Horehound (expels)

Pleurisy:

Secondary:
Angelica

Other Possible:
Elder - flower, tea
Violet - flowers, syrup

Pneumonia:

Primary:
Belladonna
Blue Vervain
Pleurisy

Secondary:
Colt's Foot
Elecampane
Ma Huang
Psyllium

Poison:

Primary:
Nettles (hemlock, henbane & belladonna)

Secondary:
Fennel - boiled in wine (vegetables)
Myrrh

Other Possible:
Arrow Root - fresh juice with water (plant)
Hops (expels)

Poison Ivy:

Secondary:
Sassafras

External:
Aloe Vera
Back Walnut
Blue Vervain
Lobelia
Sassafras
Solomon's Seal - one of the best
White Oak
Witch Hazel

Pregnancy:
See also Morning Sickness

Other Possible:
Alfalfa (good for)
Cramp Bark (pain)

Premenstrual Syndrome:

Primary:
Black Cohosh
Borage
Chamomile
Chaste Tree
Dong Quai (migraine)
False Unicorn
Pennyroyal (especially bloating)
Primrose (especially bloating)
Raspberry Leaf (cramps)
White Oak

Secondary:
Dandelion

Other Possible:
Corn silk
Sarsaparilla

Prostate:

Primary:
Saw Palmetto (all, especially enlarged)

Secondary:
Bilberry (prostatitis)
Buchu (inflammation)
Corn Silk (disorders & enlarged)
False Unicorn (disorders)
Gravel Root (inflammation)
Nettles - root
Parsley (disorders)

Other Possible:
Horsetail (disorders)
Juniper Berries (disorders)

Psoriasis:

Primary:
Oregon Grape

Secondary:
Chamomile
Milk Thistle
Sarsaparilla

External:
Aloe Vera
Black Walnut
Cayenne
Comfrey
Dong Quai
Echinacea
Gotu Kola
Lavender
Marshmallow
Milk Thistle
Oregon Grape
Poke - root
Red Clover
Sarsaparilla
Tea Tree - oil

Purgative:
See Constipation

Rabies:

Secondary:
Scullcap

Radiation Exposure:

Secondary:
Sarsaparilla (protects against)

Rash:
See Skin

Rectal:

External:
Black Pepper (prolapsed)

Rejuvenative:

Other Possible:
Gotu Kola

Relaxant:

Primary:
Lobelia
Red Clover

Reproductive Organs:

Primary:
Saw Palmetto (irritation)
Schizandra (stamina)

External:
Saw Palmetto (irritation)

Respiratory:

Primary:
Licorice (problems)
Ma Huang (complaints)
Thyme (chronic)

Restless Leg Syndrome:

Primary:
Passion Flower

Secondary:
Kava Kava
Schizandra
Valerian

Restlessness:

Primary:
Catnip
Hops
Kava Kava
Passion Flower
Sculleap

Secondary:
Butcher's Broom (restless leg syndrome)

Other Possible:
Gotu Kola

Restorative:

Other Possible:
Gotu Kola

Rheumatism:
See also Arthritis

Primary:
Alfalfa
Basil
Black Cohosh (infusion)
Blue Cohosh
Chamomile
Cramp Bark
Dandelion
Devil's Claw
Gotu Kola
Gravel Root
Guarana (headache)
Parsley
Poke - root, infused in spirits (chronic)
Sassafras - with sarsaparilla
Sculleap
Yucca (pain & inflammation)

(Rheumatism, cont'd.)

Secondary:
Allspice (pain)
Astragalus
Bilberry
Borage
Burdock
Cat's Claw
Cayenne
Centuary (muscular)
Comfrey (pain)
Hawthorne
Juniper
Kava Kava
Pau D'Arco
White Willow
Yarrow
Yerba Santa

Other Possible:
Angelica - stem juice, dried
Anise - star
Balm of Gilead
Butcher's Broom
Couch Grass
Elder - berries
Hyssop
Ma Huang
Oregon Grape
Pennyroyal
Peppermint
Pleurisy (acute & chronic)
Tea Tree

External:
Allspice - plaster, see recipe (pain)
Angelica
Arnica (pain)
Balm of Gilead - simmered with oil (pain)
Belladonna - poultice
Black Cohosh - infusion
Blue Vervain
Fennel - oil
Hops - with chamomile
Horseradish - poultice
Hyssop - leaves (muscular)
Lavender
Poke - root, extract
Rosemary - bath
Shepherd's Purse
Thyme - bath
Wormwood - oil (local anesthetic)

Rickets:

Primary:
Scullcap

Other Possible:
Horsetail

Ringworm:

External:
Black Walnut
Garlic
Golden Seal - tea, rub
Mullein - flowers
Pau D'Arco
Poke – root

River Blindness:

Primary:
Pau D'Arco

Ruptures:

Primary:
Comfrey

Saliva, Produces:

Other Possible:
Garlic
Horseradish
Nutmeg

Scalp:
See also Hair

External:
Thyme (itching)

Scarlet Fever:

Primary:
Belladonna

Other Possible:
Elder - flower

Scarring:

External:
Gotu Kola

Sciatica:

Secondary:
Burdock - tea

Scurvy:

Primary:
Dandelion
Horseradish
Shepherd's Purse

Secondary:
Bilberry - fruit
Burdock
Chickweed - juice

Other Possible:
Balm of Gilead
Barberry

Secretagogue:

Primary:
Anise

Sedative:

Primary:
Belladonna
Borage
Catnip (mild)
Chamomile
Hops
Kava Kava
Lavender
Mistletoe
Mullein
Passion Flower
Red Clover
Schizandra
Valerian
Witch Hazel

Secondary:
Primrose
Wormwood (mild)
Yarrow

Other Possible:
Hawthorne (mild)
Juniper Berries

Seizures:

Primary:
Scullcap

Senility:

Other Possible:
Gingko Biloba

Sex Drive:

Primary:
Damiana

Secondary:
Kava Kava
Nettles (men & women, diminished)
Passion Flower
Sarsaparilla (men & women)

Sexually Transmitted Diseases:

Secondary:
Sarsaparilla

Shingles:

Secondary:
Passion Flower

External:
Sarsaparilla - wash
Thyme - ointment

Shock:

Primary:
Hops

Shortness of Breath:

Secondary:
Elecampane (on exertion)

Sinusitis:
See also Congestion

Primary:
Black Cohosh
Golden Seal
Marshmallow
Thyme

Secondary:
Cayenne
Fenugreek
Garlic
Hyssop
Mullein

Other Possible:
Anise
Buchu
Horehound

External:
Eucalyptus

Skin:
See also Acne, Blemishes, Dermatitis, Pimples, Hives, Irritation & Inflammation

Primary:
Borage (healthy)
Horsetail (healthy & eliminate oil)
Oregon Grape
Primrose (disorders & health)
Raspberry Leaf (healthy)
Sassafras - with sarsaparilla (disease & purifies blood)

(Skin, cont'd.)

External:
Alfalfa (disorders)
Aloe Vera (itching, swelling, pain, scarring, wrinkles, incisions)
Agrimony (itchy)
Anise - facial pack
Arnica (irritation)
Balm of Gilead (chronic ulcers)
Basil (itchy & hives)
Belladonna (irritation)
Black Walnut
Burdock (kills streptococcus bacteria)
Centuary (spots & freckles)
Chamomile - cream (irritation, cuts, abrasions)
Coltsfoot - poultice (cooling)
Comfrey - bath (rash & dermatitis)
Dandelion (itchy)
Devil's Claw (disease)
Echinacea (wounds, sun damage)
Elder - flower, bath (soften & whiten)
Elecampane (diseases & affections)
Fennel - compress (dermatitis)
Gotu Kola (scarring)
Green Tea (wrinkles)
Henna (affections)
Honeysuckle - bark, lotion (itchy)
Hyssop - wash (irritation)
Marshmallow - bath
Mullein (softens)
Oregon Grape (heals)
Parsley (itchy)
Pennyroyal (itchy)
Poke – root, ointment - may burn slightly (diseases)
Rosemary - bath
Sarsaparilla (disease)
Senna (diseases)
Slippery Elm - poultice, one of the best (especially dry; disease, eruptions)
Solomon's Seal - distilled water (complexion)
Tea Tree - oil (dermatitis & affections)
White Oak (wounds)
White Willow - bath
Witch Hazel - tonic (wrinkles)
Yarrow (inflammation)

Sleep:
See Insomnia

Smallpox:

Primary:
Yarrow

External:
Henna

Smoking:

Primary:
Sassafras

Secondary:
Lobelia - smoke

Other Possible:
Chamomile (helps stop)

Snake Bite:

Primary:
Agrimony
Black Cohosh
Echinacea

External:
Agrimony
Black Cohosh
Black Walnut
Echinacea
Garlic

Sores:

External:
Agrimony
Blessed Thistle
Centuary (cleanses)
Chickweed - poultice (cools)
Hops
Myrrh - balm
Nettles
Sage - infusion
Solomon's Seal
White Oak

Sore Throat:
See also Throat

Primary:
Belladonna (acute)
Gotu Kola
Lobelia
Marshmallow
Slippery Elm
Thyme - infusion

Secondary:
Cayenne
Echinacea

Other Possible:
Borage

External:
Barberry - syrup
Black Walnut - gargle
Echinacea - gargle
Fenugreek - gargle
Raspberry Leaf - gargle
Sage - gargle
Thyme - gargle
White Oak - gargle
Witch Hazel

Spasms:
See Antispasmodic

Spider Bite:

External:
Tea Tree – oil

Spleen:

Primary:
Dandelion
Golden Seal

Secondary:
Fennel
Milk Thistle - infusion (obstructions, removes)
Parsley
Rhubarb

Other Possible:
Chamomile - with sugar
Honeysuckle - syrup of flowers (diseases)
Horseradish
Lavender

Sprains:

External:
Agrimony
Arnica
Comfrey
Elder - leaves, ointment
Lavender
Marshmallow
Rosemary - bath
Thyme - bath
Wormwood – poultice

Stamina:

Primary:
Astragalus
Schizandra

Staphylococcus:

Other Possible:
Golden Seal

External:
Marshmallow (sores)
St. John's Wort (sores & inflammation)
Tea Tree - oil

Stimulant:

Primary:
Aloe Vera
Angelica (aromatic)
Balm of Gilead
Bayberry
Black Pepper (mucous membrane in rectum)
Blessed Thistle
Cayenne (strong)
Cinnamon
Damiana
Dandelion
Elecampane
Eucalyptus
Frankincense
Garlic
Gravel Root
Green Tea
Guarana
Horseradish
Lavender
Myrrh
Raspberry Leaf
Rosemary
Sage
Sassafras
Tea Tree
Turmeric
Valerian
Yarrow

(Stimulant, cont'd.)

Secondary:
Anise - regular and star
Buchu (body)
Caraway
Elder - flower water (gentle)
Peppermint
Senna (slight)
Thyme
Wormwood

Other Possible:
Barberry
Cloves
Corn silk (mild)
Feverfew
Horehound (mild)
Hyssop
Pennyroyal
Shepherd's Purse

External:
Angelica (aromatic)
Bayberry - poultice with elm (indolent ulcers)
Juniper - oil (local)
Tea Tree - oil

Stomach:

Primary:
Aloe Vera (irritation)
Angelica
Barley Grass (heals)
Basil (cramps)
Cayenne
Centuary
Chamomile (nervous & cramps)
Cinnamon
Comfrey (ulcers)
Dandelion
Fenugreek
Ginger (pain)
Golden Seal
Hops
Marshmallow (inflammation)
Myrrh
Parsley (pain)
Peppermint (stomachic & abdominal cramps)

(Stomach, Primary, cont'd.)

Queen of the Meadow (disorders)
Raspberry Leaf (children)
Rhubarb
Rosemary - oil
Sage (weak)
Slippery Elm - drink, see recipe (inflammation)
Solomon's Seal - infusion (inflammation)
Witch Hazel - tea (bleeding)
Wormwood (increases activity)
Yarrow (cramps)

Secondary:
Barberry
Blessed Thistle
Blue Cohosh (cramps)
Caraway
Catnip (upset)
Ginger (pain)
Juniper - oil
Marshmallow (pain)
Pennyroyal (warming, problems with fermentation)
Thyme
Valerian
Wormwood (sickness after meals)

Other Possible:
Balm of Gilead - tincture (complaints)
Bilberry - fruit
Eyebright (stomachic)
Horseradish
Horsetail - ashes of plant, 3-10 grain (acidity)
Lavender - leaves
Mullein (cramps)
Nutmeg
Turmeric (disorders)

Stones:
See also Kidney

Primary:
Agrimony (bladder)
Corn silk
Fennel (all)

Secondary:
Milk Thistle - infusion (breaks & expels)

Stains:

External:
Shepherd's Purse - bruised herb

Strep Throat:

Secondary:
Echinacea (prevents)
Garlic
Ginger

Other Possible:
Lavender - oil

External:
Myrrh

Stress:

Primary:
Chamomile
Gotu Kola
Hops
Kava Kava
Lavender
Passion Flower
Rose Hips
Schizandra
Scullcap
Valerian

Other Possible:
Bilberry - fruit

External:
Peppermint - oil on temples

Stroke:

Primary:
Garlic (preventative)
Hawthorne

Secondary:
Gingko Biloba

Sunburn:

External:
Aloe Vera
Balm of Gilead - simmered with oil
Chamomile
Comfrey
Echinacea (sun damage)
Witch Hazel (inflammation)

Swelling:

Secondary:
Hawthorne (ankles)

External:
Arnica (reduces)
Balm of Gilead - with lard or oil
Borage - poultice
Chamomile (joint)
Comfrey
Myrrh
Parsley - poultice
Slippery Elm - poultice
St. John's Wort
Thyme - ointment or bath
Violet - leaves, plaster & poultice
Witch Hazel
Wormwood - poultice
Yerba Santa - poultice

Syphilis:

Primary:
Echinacea
Sassafras - with sarsaparilla

Secondary:
Burdock
Butchers Broom
Oregon Grape
Sarsaparilla
Other Possible:
Dragon's Blood
Elder - berries
Lobelia
Yerba Santa

External:
Golden Seal

Tapeworm:
See also Worms

Primary:
Slippery Elm - with oil of male fern

Secondary:
Poke – root

Teeth:
See also Dental Problems

Primary:
Horsetail (strengthens)
Raspberry Leaf (healthy)

Secondary:
Thyme

Other Possible:
Marshmallow

External:
Alfalfa (decaying)
Chamomile
Myrrh (decay)
Peppermint (pain & cavities)
Sage - brush
Thyme - oil, paste & mouthwash
White Oak
Witch Hazel

Tendonitis:

Primary:
Devil's Claw (pain)

Tension:

Primary:
Lady's Slipper
Lavender
Valerian

Secondary:
Black Cohosh

Other Possible:
Feverfew

Testis:

Other Possible:
Chickweed (swollen)

Tetanus:

Primary:
Lobelia

Thirst:

Secondary:
Licorice (prevents, excellent)

External:
Yerba Santa - chew

Throat:
See also Sore Throat

Primary:
Licorice (sore)
Pleurisy (catarrh)
Slippery Elm (sore)

Secondary:
Elder - flower, hot tea at bedtime (problems)
Mullein (inflammation)

Other Possible:
Centuary (sore)
Hawthorne (sore)
Horehound
Marshmallow
Psyllium (sore)
Yerba Santa (irritation)

External:
Bayberry - gargle (inflammation, chronic)
Bilberry - leaves & bark (ulceration)
Honey Suckle - bark, gargle
Hyssop (sore)
Sage - gargle (inflamed)
Tea Tree – oil, gargle with water

Thrush:

External:
Myrrh

Thyroid:

Primary:
Bladderwrack (stimulant)
Parsley

Tissue:

Primary:
Gotu Kola
Shepherd's Purse (contracts)
Secondary:
Lady's Mantle (contracts)

Other Possible:
Chamomile
Coltsfoot (promotes healing)

Tonic:

Primary:
Barberry (blood)
Blessed Thistle - cold infusion
Borage (adrenal)
Catnip
Centuary
Chamomile
Damiana (general)
Eyebright (slight)
Golden Seal
Mistletoe
Myrrh
Oregon Grape
Rosemary
Sage
Solomon's Seal
Thyme
White Willow
Witch Hazel
Wormwood
Yarrow
Yerba Santa

Secondary:
Alfalfa (overall)
Angelica (infusion)
Coltsfoot
Elecampane
False Unicorn
Guarana
Horehound
Licorice

Other Possible:
Balm of Gilead
Bayberry
Dong Quai
Hawthorne
Horseradish
Pleurisy
Queen of the Meadow
Scullcap
Valerian

Tonsillitis:

Primary:
Gotu Kola

Secondary:
Burdock
Sage

Other Possible:
Wormwood (inflammation)

External:
Sage – gargle

Toothache:

Primary:
Hops
White Willow

External:
Caraway - oil soaked on cotton
Chamomile - wash
Cloves - oil
Echinacea
Kava Kava
Lavender
Witch Hazel
Yarrow

Tooth Decay:
See Teeth

Toxins:

Other Possible:
Myrrh (prevents absorption)

Tranquilizer:

Primary:
Chamomile
Mistletoe

Secondary:
St. John's Wort

Other Possible:
Blue Vervain - with mistletoe

Tuberculosis:

Primary:
Comfrey
Red Clover

Other Possible:
Garlic

Typhoid Fever:

Primary:
Belladonna
Sage - tea
Slippery Elm - compound, see recipe

Secondary:
Agrimony

Other Possible:
Angelica
Barberry
Boneset
Oregon Grape (early stages)

Ulcers:

Primary:
Alfalfa (peptic)
Barley Grass (duodenal)
Cat's Claw
Cayenne

(Ulcers, Primary, cont'd.)

Chamomile (peptic, prevent & treat)
Comfrey (internal especially liver & peptic)
Garlic (peptic)
Golden Seal - with myrrh, one of the best
Hops
Licorice (peptic)
Marshmallow (peptic)
Myrrh - with golden seal, one of the best
Pau D'Arco (peptic & gastric)
Rhubarb (duodenal)
Valerian
Yarrow

Secondary:
Agrimony
Aloe Vera (peptic)
Barberry (kills bacteria that cause peptic)
Bilberry (peptic)
Cinnamon (peptic)
Frankincense
Horsetail
Peppermint (peptic)
Psyllium (peptic)
Slippery Elm
St. John's Wort

Other Possible:
Bayberry
Coltsfoot

External:
Balm of Gilead (chronic skin)
Bilberry - leaves & bark
Black Walnut
Borage - gargle (mouth)
Centuary (closes)
Chickweed - poultice (indolent)
Golden Seal
Lobelia - poultice
Myrrh - tincture
Raspberry Leaf - wash
Rhubarb
Sarsaparilla - wash (indolent)
Slippery Elm - poultice, one of the best
White Oak - poultice

Urinary Tract:

See also Infections

Primary:

Bilberry - fruit (complaints)
Butcher's Broom (obstructions)
Sarsaparilla (disorders)

Secondary:

Angelica (diseases)
Balm of Gilead (diseases)
Black Pepper (stimulates)
Corn Silk (mucus in urine)
Couch Grass (diseases & inflammation)
Damiana (infections)
Horsetail (ulcers)
Kava Kava - (infection & pain)

Urine Suppression:

Primary:

St. John's Wort

Uterus:

Primary:

Nettles (tonic)
Raspberry Leaf (strengthens & spasms)

Secondary:

Shepherd's Purse (tones & returns to normal size after childbirth)

Other Possible:

Cramp Bark
Scullcap (relaxer)

Vaginal Dryness:

Primary:

Dong Quai

External:

Aloe Vera

Vaginitis:

Primary:

Blue Cohosh
Kava Kava

Secondary:

Garlic

External:

Tea Tree - oil
Witch Hazel - douche
Yarrow

Varicose Veins:

Primary:

Butcher's Broom
White Oak

Secondary:

Hawthorne
Witch Hazel

External:

Bayberry (discomfort & swelling)
Butcher's Broom - cream (during pregnancy)
Comfrey - compress
Rosemary - bath
Witch Hazel

Vertigo:

Secondary:

Gingko Biloba
Lavender
Pennyroyal

Other Possible:

Black Pepper
Blessed Thistle
Butcher's Broom

Viral Infection:

See Antiviral & Infection

Vomiting:

Primary:

Basil - infusion
Cinnamon
Cloves - oil, 2 drops in 1-cup water
Fennel
Ginger (all, especially after surgery or chemotherapy)
Golden Seal
Lady's Mantle (blood)
Peppermint - oil
Slippery Elm (pain after)

Secondary:

Frankincense
Nutmeg
St. John's Wort
White Oak

Other Possible:

Lavender - leaves
Yerba Santa

Warts:

External:

Basil - seeds
Black Walnut
Chickweed
Comfrey
Dandelion - sap
Garlic
Mullein
Pau D'Arco
Tea Tree - oil
Thyme - ointment

Weakness:

Secondary:

Chaste Tree

Weaning:

Primary:

Arrowroot

Weight – Increases:

Other Possible:

Alfalfa - infusion, 1 ounce to 1 pint in cupful doses

Wheezing:

Primary:

Feverfew - with honey

Secondary:

Coltsfoot - juice or syrup
Fennel
Horehound – syrup

Whooping Cough:

Primary:

Black Cohosh
Comfrey
Elecampane
Horseradish - with vinegar & glycerin
Marshmallow - see recipe
Pennyroyal - 1 spoon juice with sugar
Red Clover - infusion
Thyme - fresh

Secondary:

Violet - leaves

Other Possible:

Mullein
Primrose

Worms:

Primary:
Aloe Vera (internal)
Black Walnut (expels)
Blue Vervain
Boneset (intestinal)
Chamomile
Feverfew
Horseradish - one of the best
Nettles
Parsley
St. John's Wort (intestinal)
White Willow

Secondary:
Bladderwrack
Blessed Thistle - powdered leaves
Centuary
False Unicorn
Horehound - powdered leaves (destroys & expels)
Lady's Slipper
Myrrh
Poke - root (tapeworm)
Rhubarb (especially thread worms)
Senna - following wormwood
Thyme (intestinal)

Other Possible:
Lobelia
Tea Tree (especially round worms)

External:
Black Walnut (on lawns)

Wounds:

Primary:
Lady's Mantle - decoction, one of the best (internal)

External:
Agrimony
Aloe Vera
Arnica (promotes healing)
Balm of Gilead (infected)
Black Walnut
Blue Vervain - poultice
Centuary
Comfrey (heals)
Dandelion
Dragons Blood
Elder - leaves & flowers, ointment
Golden Seal
Gotu Kola
Horsetail - poultice (bleeding)
Hyssop
Juniper - oil mixed with lard (animals)
Lady's Mantle - one of the best (dries up deep wounds & promotes cell growth)
Lavender
Marshmallow (discharges)
Mullein
Myrrh
Pau D'Arco
Raspberry Leaf - wash
Red Clover (mucous)
Rosemary
Sarsaparilla
Shepherd's Purse (bleeding)
Slippery Elm - poultice, one of the best
Solomon's Seal
St. John's Wort - compress
Tea Tree - oil (disinfects)
White Oak (skin)
Witch Hazel (small)
Yarrow - poultice (discharges)

Yeast:

See also Infections

Primary:

Garlic
Pau D'Arco

Secondary:

Echinacea
Garlic

External:

Barberry
Garlic (inhibits)
Nettles
Pau D'Arco
Tea Tree - oil, douche with water
Thyme

Yellow Fever:

Other Possible:

Boneset

Bibliography

Balch, CNC, Phyllis A. Prescription for Herbal Healing. New York: Avery Books, member of Penguin Putman Inc., 2002

Balch, CNC, Phyllis A. and James F. Balch, M.D. Prescription for Nutritional Healing. 3rd Edition. New York: Avery Books, member of Penguin Putman Inc., 2000

Balch, CNC, Phyllis A. and James F. Balch, M.D. Prescription for Nutritional Healing. 4th Edition. New York: Avery Books, member of Penguin Putman Inc., 2006

Blose, Nora and Dawn Cusick. Herb Drying Handbook. New York: Sterling Publishing Company, Inc., 1993

Cunningham, Scott. Cunningham's Encyclopedia of Magical Herbs. Minnesota: Llewellyn Publications, 1993

Grieve, Mrs. M. A Modern Herbal, Volume I, A-H. New York: Dover, 1971. New York: Harcourt, Brace and Company, 1931

Grieve, Mrs. M. A Modern Herbal, Volume II, I-Z. New York: Dover, 1971. New York: Harcourt, Brace and Company, 1931

Hedley, Christopher and Non Shaw. Herbal Remedies, A Practical Beginner's Guide to Making Effective Remedies in the Kitchen. New York: Smithmark Publishers, 1996

Mindell R. Ph, Ph.D, Earl and Carol Coleman. Earl Mindell's Herb Bible. New York: Simon and Schuster / Fireside, 1992

Parvati, Jeannine. Hygieia, A Woman's Herbal. Firestone Collective, 1978

Rose, Jeanne. Herbs & Things. New York: Putnam Publishing Group, 1972

Ryall, Rhiannon. The Magic of Herbs. Berks, United Kingdom, 1996

Shepherd, James. (herbalist, occultist), in discussion with author, 1990 – 2008

The Goddess Tree. August 2008. Gwendolyn. December 2007 – September 2008. http://thegoddesstree.ning.com

Weiner, Dr. Michael A. The Herbal Bible. California: Quantum Books, 1992

Photo Bibliography

Photography used in illustrations: (Photographers and artists do not endorse the use of the following herbs or the content of this book.)

Agrimony: Photography by Pethan July 26, 2005, under the terms of the GNU Free Documentation License, and the Creative Commons Attribution-Share Alike 3.0 Unported license.
http://commons.wikimedia.org/wiki/File:Agrimonia_eupatoria01.jpg

Alfalfa: Karen Bergeron and Alternative Nature Enterprises, PO Box 221 Tennessee Ridge TN 37178 email karen@altnature.com.
http://www.freeherbpictures.com/alfalfa-herb-pictures.htm

Angelica: Karen Bergeron and Alternative Nature Enterprises, PO Box 221 Tennessee Ridge TN 37178 email karen@altnature.com.
http://www.freeherbpictures.com/angelica-herb-pictures.htm

Anise: Photography by FASTILY August 3, 2009, under the terms of the GNU Free Documentation License, and the Creative Commons Attribution-Share Alike 3.0 Unported license.
http://commons.wikimedia.org/wiki/File:Anise3300ppx.jpg

Anise, Star: Photography by MarkSweep March 18, 2005, under the terms of the GNU Free Documentation License, and the Creative Commons Attribution-Share Alike 3.0 Unported license.
http://commons.wikimedia.org/wiki/File:StarAnise.jpg

Arnica: Karen Bergeron and Alternative Nature Enterprises, PO Box 221 Tennessee Ridge TN 37178 email karen@altnature.com.
http://www.freeherbpictures.com/arnica-herb-pictures.htm

Arrowroot: Photography by Challiyan August 5, 2008, under the terms of the GNU Free Documentation License, and the Creative Commons Attribution-Share Alike 3.0 Unported license.
http://commons.wikimedia.org/wiki/File:Arrowroot_flower.jpg

Astragalus: Photography by Doronenko June 24, 2007, under the terms of the GNU Free Documentation License, and the Creative Commons Attribution-Share Alike 3.0 Unported license.
http://commons.wikimedia.org/wiki/File:Astragalus_membranaceus.jpg

Barberry: Photography by Teun Spaans April 30, 2007, under the terms of the GNU Free Documentation License, and the Creative Commons Attribution-Share Alike 3.0 Unported license.
http://commons.wikimedia.org/wiki/File:Zuurbes_R0021693.JPG

Barley Grass: Photography by Topjabot October 27, 2004, under the terms of the GNU Free Documentation License, and the Creative Commons Attribution-Share Alike 3.0 Unported license.
http://commons.wikimedia.org/wiki/File:Hordeum_distichon0.jpg

Basil: Karen Bergeron and Alternative Nature Enterprises, PO Box 221 Tennessee Ridge TN 37178 email karen@altnature.com.
http://www.freeherbpictures.com/basil-herb-pictures.htm

Bayberry: Photography by Fepup May 24, 2009, under Public Domain.
http://commons.wikimedia.org/wiki/File:Myrica_cerifera_1.JPG

Belladonna: Photography of berry by Topjabot October 26, 2004, under the terms of the GNU Free Documentation License, and the Creative Commons Attribution-Share Alike 3.0 Unported license.
http://commons.wikimedia.org/wiki/File:Atropa_bella-donna0.jpg
Photography of flower by BerndH June 22, 2005, under the terms of the GNU Free Documentation License, and the Creative Commons Attribution-Share Alike 3.0 Unported license.
http://commons.wikimedia.org/wiki/File:Atropa_belladonna_220605.jpg

Bilberry: Photography by Banangraut October 14, 2006, under the terms of the GNU Free Documentation License, and the Creative Commons Attribution-Share Alike 3.0 Unported license.
http://commons.wikimedia.org/wiki/File:Bl%C3%A5b%C3%A6r_1.jpg

Black Cohosh: Karen Bergeron and Alternative Nature Enterprises, PO Box 221 Tennessee Ridge TN 37178 email karen@altnature.com.
http://www.freeherbpictures.com/black-cohosh-pictures.htm

Black Pepper: Photography by Antti Kivivalli March 12, 2007, under the terms of the GNU Free Documentation License, and the Creative Commons Attribution-Share Alike 3.0 Unported license.
http://commons.wikimedia.org/wiki/File:Peppercorn.jpg

Black Walnut: Photography by MONGO August 20, 2006, under Public Domain.
http://commons.wikimedia.org/wiki/File:Black_Walnut_nut_and_leave_detail.JPG

Bladderwrack: Photography by EvaK November 13, 2006, under the terms of the GNU Free Documentation License, and the Creative Commons Attribution-Share Alike 3.0 Unported license.
http://commons.wikimedia.org/wiki/File:Fucus_vesiculosus_Wales.jpg

Blessed Thistle: Photography by http://www.pharmazie.uni-mainz.de/AK-Stoe/DB/Gruppe05/cnicus_benedictus.htm. No listed copyright.

Blue Cohosh: Photography by H. Zell August 27, 2009, (fruit), April 29, 2009, (plant) under the terms of the GNU Free Documentation License, and the Creative Commons Attribution-Share Alike 3.0 Unported license.
http://commons.wikimedia.org/wiki/File:Caulophyllum_thalictroides_003.JPG

Blue Vervain: Karen Bergeron and Alternative Nature Enterprises, PO Box 221 Tennessee Ridge TN 37178 email karen@altnature.com.
http://www.freeherbpictures.com/blue-vervain-herb-pictures.htm

Boneset: Photography by H. Zell July 16, 2009, under the terms of the GNU Free Documentation License, and the Creative Commons Attribution-Share Alike 3.0 Unported license.
http://commons.wikimedia.org/wiki/File:Eupatorium_perfoliatum_0003.JPG

Borage: Karen Bergeron and Alternative Nature Enterprises, PO Box 221 Tennessee Ridge TN 37178 email karen@altnature.com.
http://www.freeherbpictures.com/borage-herb-pictures.htm

Burdock: Photography by Christian Fischer July 30, 2008, under the terms of the GNU Free Documentation License, and the Creative Commons Attribution-Share Alike 3.0 Unported license.
http://commons.wikimedia.org/wiki/File:ArctiumLappa4.jpg

Butcher's Broom: Photography by Hans Hillewaert April 2, 2008, under the terms of the GNU Free Documentation License, and the Creative Commons Attribution-Share Alike 3.0 Unported license.
http://commons.wikimedia.org/wiki/File:Ruscus_aculeatus.jpg

Caraway: Photography by H. Zell May 9, 2010, under the terms of the GNU Free Documentation License, and the Creative Commons Attribution-Share Alike 3.0 Unported license.
http://commons.wikimedia.org/wiki/File:Carum_carvi_002.JPG

Catnip: Karen Bergeron and Alternative Nature Enterprises, PO Box 221 Tennessee Ridge TN 37178 email karen@altnature.com.
http://www.freeherbpictures.com/catnip-herb-pictures.htm

Cat's Claw: Photography by Johannes Keplinger April 4, 2006, under the terms of the GNU Free Documentation License, and the Creative Commons Attribution-Share Alike 3.0 Unported license.
http://commons.wikimedia.org/wiki/File:Thorns_U_tomentosa.jpg

Centuary: Photography by Hans Hillewaert June 30, 2006, under the terms of the GNU Free Documentation License, and the Creative Commons Attribution-Share Alike 3.0 Unported license.
http://commons.wikimedia.org/wiki/File:Centaurium_erythraea_(flowers).jpg

Chamomile: Photography by H. Zell September 27, 2009, under the terms of the GNU Free Documentation License, and the Creative Commons Attribution-Share Alike 3.0 Unported license.
http://commons.wikimedia.org/wiki/File:Matricaria_recutita_003.JPG

Chaste Tree: Photography by H. Zell August 12, 2009, under the terms of the GNU Free Documentation License, and the Creative Commons Attribution-Share Alike 3.0 Unported license.
http://commons.wikimedia.org/wiki/File:Vitex_agnus-castus_002.JPG
http://commons.wikimedia.org/wiki/File:Vitex_agnus-castus_003.JPG

Chickweed: Photography by Rasbak under the terms of the GNU Free Documentation License, and the Creative Commons Attribution-Share Alike 3.0 Unported license.
http://commons.wikimedia.org/wiki/File:Stellaria_media_(vogelmuur).jpg

Cinnamon: Photography by MPF February 7, 2006, under Public Domain in the United States because it is a work of the United States Federal Government under the terms of Title 17, Chapter 1, Section 105 of the US Code.
http://commons.wikimedia.org/wiki/File:Cinnamomum_verum1.jpg

Coltsfoot: Photography by H. Zell April 8, 2009, under the terms of the GNU Free Documentation License, and the Creative Commons Attribution-Share Alike 3.0 Unported license.
http://commons.wikimedia.org/wiki/File:Tussilago_farfara_002.JPG

Comfrey: Karen Bergeron and Alternative Nature Enterprises, PO Box 221 Tennessee Ridge TN 37178 email karen@altnature.com.
http://www.freeherbpictures.com/comfrey-herb-pictures.htm

Corn Silk: Photography by H. Zell July 16, 2009, under the terms of the GNU Free Documentation License, and the Creative Commons Attribution-Share Alike 3.0 Unported license.
http://commons.wikimedia.org/wiki/File:Zea_mays_003.JPG

Cramp Bark: Photography by Arnstein Rønning June 11, 2009, under the terms of the GNU Free Documentation License, and the Creative Commons Attribution-Share Alike 3.0 Unported license.

http://commons.wikimedia.org/wiki/File:Viburnum_opulus_.JPG

Berries by Texnik August 2008 under the terms of the GNU Free Documentation License, and the Creative Commons Attribution-Share Alike 3.0 Unported license.

http://commons.wikimedia.org/wiki/File:Viburnum_opulus_-_kalyna_ukraine.jpg

Damiana: Photography by H. Zell May 8, 2010, under the terms of the GNU Free Documentation License, and the Creative Commons Attribution-Share Alike 3.0 Unported license.

http://commons.wikimedia.org/wiki/File:Turnera_diffusa_var._aphrodisiaca_002.JPG

Dandelion: Karen Bergeron and Alternative Nature Enterprises, PO Box 221 Tennessee Ridge TN 37178 email karen@altnature.com.

http://www.freeherbpictures.com/dandelion-herb-pictures.htm

Devil's Claw: Photography by Henri Pidoux December 16, 2005, under under the terms of the GNU Free Documentation License, and the Creative Commons Attribution-Share Alike 3.0 Unported license.

http://commons.wikimedia.org/wiki/File:Harpagophytum_5.jpg

Dong Quai: Karen Bergeron and Alternative Nature Enterprises, PO Box 221 Tennessee Ridge TN 37178 email karen@altnature.com.

http://www.freeherbpictures.com/don-quai-herb-pictures.htm

Dragon's Blood: Photography by Sezohanim 2008, under the terms of the GNU Free Documentation License, and the Creative Commons Attribution-Share Alike 3.0 Unported license.

http://creativecommons.org/licenses/by/2.0/deed.en

Echinacea: Photography by H. Zell July 16, 2009, under the terms of the GNU Free Documentation License, and the Creative Commons Attribution-Share Alike 3.0 Unported license.

http://commons.wikimedia.org/wiki/File:Echinacea_purpurea_002.JPG

Elder: Karen Bergeron and Alternative Nature Enterprises (flowers), PO Box 221 Tennessee Ridge TN 37178 email karen@altnature.com.

http://www.freeherbpictures.com/elder-flowers-pictures.htm

Berries: Photography by Nova February 8, 2005, under the terms of the GNU Free Documentation License, and the Creative Commons Attribution-Share Alike 3.0 Unported license.

http://commons.wikimedia.org/wiki/File:Sambucus_nigra2.jpg

Elecampane: Photography by H. Zell June 9, 2009, under the terms of the GNU Free Documentation License, and the Creative Commons Attribution-Share Alike 3.0 Unported license.

http://commons.wikimedia.org/wiki/File:Inula_helenium_003.JPG

Eucalyptus: Photography by Forest & Kim Starr November 23, 2005, under the terms of the GNU Free Documentation License, and the Creative Commons Attribution-Share Alike 3.0 Unported license.

http://commons.wikimedia.org/wiki/File:Starr_051123-5467_Eucalyptus_globulus.jpg

Eyebright: Photography by Rasbak January 11, 2005, under the terms of the GNU Free Documentation License, and the Creative Commons Attribution-Share Alike 3.0 Unported license.

http://commons.wikimedia.org/wiki/File:Augentrost.jpg

False Unicorn: Photography by Phyzome June 2, 2005, under the terms of the GNU Free Documentation License, and the Creative Commons Attribution-Share Alike 3.0 Unported license.
http://commons.wikimedia.org/wiki/File:Chamaelirium_luteum_-_false_unicorn_-_desc-flowering_heads_closed.jpg

Fennel: Photography by H. Zell July 16, 2009, under the terms of the GNU Free Documentation License, and the Creative Commons Attribution-Share Alike 3.0 Unported license.
http://commons.wikimedia.org/wiki/File:Foeniculum_vulgare_003.JPG

Feverfew: Photography by Steffen Heinz Caronna under the terms of the GNU Free Documentation License, and the Creative Commons Attribution-Share Alike 3.0 Unported license.
http://commons.wikimedia.org/wiki/File:Tanacetum_parthenium_Bl%C3%BCten.JPG

Garlic: Photography by Kickof July 7, 2009, under the terms of the GNU Free Documentation License, and the Creative Commons Attribution-Share Alike 3.0 Unported license.
http://commons.wikimedia.org/wiki/File:Knoblauch_Bluete_3.JPG

Ginger: Photography by Dalgial September 10, 2009, under the terms of the GNU Free Documentation License, and the Creative Commons Attribution-Share Alike 3.0 Unported license.
http://commons.wikimedia.org/wiki/File:Zingiber_officinale.JPG

Gingko Biloba: Photography by H. Zell October 3, 2010, under the terms of the GNU Free Documentation License, and the Creative Commons Attribution-Share Alike 3.0 Unported license.
http://commons.wikimedia.org/wiki/File:Ginkgo_biloba_010.JPG

Golden Seal: Photography by James Steakley May 17, 2009, under the terms of the GNU Free Documentation License, and the Creative Commons Attribution-Share Alike 3.0 Unported license.
http://commons.wikimedia.org/wiki/File:Hydrastis.jpg

Gotu Kola: Photography by Forest & Kim Starr August 3, 2002, under the terms of the GNU Free Documentation License, and the Creative Commons Attribution-Share Alike 3.0 Unported license.
http://commons.wikimedia.org/wiki/File:Starr_020803-0094_Centella_asiatica.jpg

Gravel Root: Photography by Jarekt July 9, 2008, under the terms of the GNU Free Documentation License, and the Creative Commons Attribution-Share Alike 3.0 Unported license.
http://commons.wikimedia.org/wiki/File:Eupatorium-purpureum2.JPG

Green Tea: Photography by Qwert1234 October 9, 2009, under Public Domain.
http://commons.wikimedia.org/wiki/File:Camellia_sinensis_Japan.JPG

Guarana: Photography by Denis Barthel March 2004, under the terms of the GNU Free Documentation License, and the Creative Commons Attribution-Share Alike 3.0 Unported license.
http://commons.wikimedia.org/wiki/File:Guarana_-_Paullinia_cupana.jpg

Hawthorne: Photography by Sten Porse October 5, 2007, under the terms of the GNU Free Documentation License, and the Creative Commons Attribution-Share Alike 3.0 Unported license.
http://commons.wikimedia.org/wiki/File:Crataegus-oxyacantha-flowers.JPG

Hemlock (Wood): Photography by MPF August 12, 2009, and is a work of the Natural Resources Conservation Service, part of the United States Department of Agriculture, taken or made during the course of an employee's official duties. As a work of the U.S. federal government, the image is in the public domain.

http://commons.wikimedia.org/wiki/File:Conium_maculatum.jpg

Hemlock (Water): Photography by Kristian Peters June 28, 2006, under the terms of the GNU Free Documentation License, and the Creative Commons Attribution-Share Alike 3.0 Unported license.

http://commons.wikimedia.org/wiki/File:Cicuta_virosa.jpeg

Hemp: Photography by United States Fish and Wildlife Service August 1, 2007, and is the work of a U.S. Fish and Wildlife Service employee, taken or made during the course of an employee's official duties. As a work of the U.S. federal government, the image is in the public domain.

http://commons.wikimedia.org/wiki/File:Marijuana.jpg

Honeysuckle: Photography by Robert Flogaus-Faust May 23, 2009, under the terms of the GNU Free Documentation License, and the Creative Commons Attribution-Share Alike 3.0 Unported license.

http://commons.wikimedia.org/wiki/File:Lonicera_caprifolium_RF.jpg

Hops: Photography by Lestat (Jan Mehlich) August 29, 2007, under the terms of the GNU Free Documentation License, and the Creative Commons Attribution-Share Alike 3.0 Unported license.

http://commons.wikimedia.org/wiki/File:Chmiel_zwyczajny_-_szyszka.JPG

Horehound: Photography by Eugene Zelenko Feburary 24, 2007, under the terms of the GNU Free Documentation License, and the Creative Commons Attribution-Share Alike 3.0 Unported license.

http://commons.wikimedia.org/wiki/File:Marrubium_vulgare2.jpg

Horseradish: Photography by Sanja565658 August 24, 2009, under the terms of the GNU Free Documentation License, and the Creative Commons Attribution-Share Alike 3.0 Unported license.

http://commons.wikimedia.org/wiki/File:Armoracia_rusticana_01.JPG

Horsetail: Photography by Kropsoq May 2005, under the terms of the GNU Free Documentation License, and the Creative Commons Attribution-Share Alike 3.0 Unported license.

http://commons.wikimedia.org/wiki/File:Equisetum_arvense_2005_spring_002.jpg

Hyssop: Photography by Photography by H. Zell June 27, 2009, under the terms of the GNU Free Documentation License, and the Creative Commons Attribution-Share Alike 3.0 Unported license.

http://commons.wikimedia.org/wiki/File:Hyssopus_officinalis_005.JPG

Juniper: Photography by Stan Shebs September 24, 2006, under the terms of the GNU Free Documentation License, and the Creative Commons Attribution-Share Alike 3.0 Unported license.

http://commons.wikimedia.org/wiki/File:Juniperus_communis_var_depressa_5.jpg

Kava Kava: Photography by Forest & Kim Starr March 18, 2004, under the terms of the GNU Free Documentation License, and the Creative Commons Attribution-Share Alike 3.0 Unported license.

http://commons.wikimedia.org/wiki/File:Starr_040318-0058_Piper_methysticum.jpg

Lady's Mantle: Photography by Jina Lee April 28, 2007, under the terms of the GNU Free Documentation License, and the Creative Commons Attribution-Share Alike 3.0 Unported license.
http://commons.wikimedia.org/wiki/File:Lady%27s_Mantle_Alchemilla_vulgaris_2816px.jpg

Lady's Slipper: Photography by July 4, 2010, under the terms of the GNU Free Documentation License, and the Creative Commons Attribution-Share Alike 3.0 Unported license.
http://commons.wikimedia.org/wiki/File:Yellow_Lady%27s-slipper,_Port_aux_Choix,_NL.jpg

Lavender: Photography by Off2riorob July 2010, under the terms of the GNU Free Documentation License, and the Creative Commons Attribution-Share Alike 3.0 Unported license.
http://commons.wikimedia.org/wiki/File:Lavender.JPG

Lobelia: Photography by H. Zell July 29, 2009, under the terms of the GNU Free Documentation License, and the Creative Commons Attribution-Share Alike 3.0 Unported license.
http://commons.wikimedia.org/wiki/File:Lobelia_inflata_003.JPG

Marshmallow: Photography by H. Zell July 16, 2009, under the terms of the GNU Free Documentation License, and the Creative Commons Attribution-Share Alike 3.0 Unported license.
http://commons.wikimedia.org/wiki/File:Althaea_officinalis_003.JPG

Milk Thistle: Photography by H. Zell July 8, 2009, under the terms of the GNU Free Documentation License, and the Creative Commons Attribution-Share Alike 3.0 Unported license.
http://commons.wikimedia.org/wiki/File:Silybum_marianum_0003.JPG

Mistletoe: Photography by H. Zell November 15, 2009, under the terms of the GNU Free Documentation License, and the Creative Commons Attribution-Share Alike 3.0 Unported license.
http://commons.wikimedia.org/wiki/File:Viscum_album_002.JPG

Mullein: Photography by Stan Shebs June 11, 2006, under the terms of the GNU Free Documentation License, and the Creative Commons Attribution-Share Alike 3.0 Unported license.
http://commons.wikimedia.org/wiki/File:Verbascum_thapsus_4.jpg

Nettles: Photography by G.dallorto February 20, 2006. The copyright holder of this file allows anyone to use it for any purpose, provided that the copyright holder is properly attributed. Redistribution, derivative work, commercial use, and all other use is permitted.
http://commons.wikimedia.org/wiki/File:Nettle_-_Ortica_-_Foto_Giovanni_Dall%27Orto.jpg

Nutmeg: Photography by W.A. Djatmiko January 12, 2008, under the terms of the GNU Free Documentation License, and the Creative Commons Attribution-Share Alike 3.0 Unported license.
http://commons.wikimedia.org/wiki/File:Myris_fragr_Fr_080112-3290_ltn.jpg

Oregon Grape: Photography by Kurt Stueber October 27, 2004, under the terms of the GNU Free Documentation License, and the Creative Commons Attribution-Share Alike 3.0 Unported license.
http://commons.wikimedia.org/wiki/File:Mahonia_aquifolium0.jpg

Parsley: Photography by H. Zell October 24, 2009, under the terms of the GNU Free Documentation License, and the Creative Commons Attribution-Share Alike 3.0 Unported license.
http://commons.wikimedia.org/wiki/File:Petroselinum_crispum_003.JPG

Passion Flower: Photography by Mark Cooper 1997, specifically for this publication. No copyright.
http://members.aol.com/pasiflora1

Pau D'Arco: Photography by Carla Antonini August 17, 2006, under the Creative Commons Attribution-Share Alike 2.5 Argentina license.
http://commons.wikimedia.org/wiki/File:Tabebuia_impetiginosa_inflorescencias.jpeg

Pennyroyal: Photography by H. Zell August 4, 2009, under the terms of the GNU Free Documentation License, and the Creative Commons Attribution-Share Alike 3.0 Unported license.
http://commons.wikimedia.org/wiki/File:Mentha_pulegium_003.JPG

Peppermint: Photography by Angela May 31, 2004, and is in the public domain because it contains materials that originally came from the Agricultural Research Service, the research agency of the United States Department of Agriculture.
http://commons.wikimedia.org/wiki/File:Peppermint_and_Corsican_mint_plant_shorter.jpg

Pleurisy: Photography by H. Zell June 17, 2009, under the terms of the GNU Free Documentation License, and the Creative Commons Attribution-Share Alike 3.0 Unported license.
http://commons.wikimedia.org/wiki/File:Asclepias_tuberosa_002.JPG

Primrose: Photography by TeunSpaans July 5, 2005, under the terms of the GNU Free Documentation License, and the Creative Commons Attribution-Share Alike 3.0 Unported license.
http://commons.wikimedia.org/wiki/File:Middelste_teunis_bloem_R0011876.JPG

Psyllium: Photography by Aroche August 21, 2006, under the terms of the GNU Free Documentation License, and the Creative Commons Attribution-Share Alike 2.5 Unported license.
http://commons.wikimedia.org/wiki/File:Plantago_scabra2.jpg

Queen of the Meadow: Photography by H. Zell June 9, 2009, under the terms of the GNU Free Documentation License, and the Creative Commons Attribution-Share Alike 3.0 Unported license.
http://commons.wikimedia.org/wiki/File:Filipendula_ulmaria_003.JPG

Raspberry: Photography by Juhanson June 27, 2005, under the terms of the GNU Free Documentation License, and the Creative Commons Attribution-Share Alike 3.0 Unported license.
http://commons.wikimedia.org/wiki/File:Raspberries_(Rubus_Idaeus).jpg

Red Clover: Photography by H. Zell May 2, 2009, under the terms of the GNU Free Documentation License, and the Creative Commons Attribution-Share Alike 3.0 Unported license.
http://commons.wikimedia.org/wiki/File:Trifolium_pratense_002.JPG

Rhubarb: Photography by Wouter Hagens May 11, 2005, under Public Domain.
http://commons.wikimedia.org/wiki/File:Rheum_rhaponticum_A.jpg

Rose Hips: Photography by VoDeTan2March 15, 2010, under the terms of the GNU Free Documentation License, and the Creative Commons Attribution-Share Alike 2.5 Unported license.
http://commons.wikimedia.org/wiki/File:Crataegus_pedicellata.jpg

Rosemary: Photography by Luigi Chiesa April 22, 2006, under the terms of the GNU Free Documentation License, and the Creative Commons Attribution-Share Alike 3.0 Unported license.
http://commons.wikimedia.org/wiki/File:Rosmarino_fiori.jpg

Sage: Photography by David Monniaux January 1, 2007, under the terms of the GNU Free Documentation License, and the Creative Commons Attribution-Share Alike 3.0 Unported license.
http://commons.wikimedia.org/wiki/File:Salvia_officinalis_p1150381.jpg
Flower by Wildfeuer October 20, 2006 under the terms of the GNU Free Documentation License, and the Creative Commons Attribution-Share Alike 3.0 Unported license.
http://commons.wikimedia.org/wiki/File:2006-10-30-Salvia03.jpg

Sassafras: Photography by Rlevse May 22, 2010, under the terms of the GNU Free Documentation License, and the Creative Commons Attribution-Share Alike 3.0 Unported license.
http://commons.wikimedia.org/wiki/File:Sassafras_albidum_3_lobe_variations_B.JPG

Saw Palmetto: Photography by H. Zell July 29, 2009, under the terms of the GNU Free Documentation License, and the Creative Commons Attribution-Share Alike 3.0 Unported license.
http://commons.wikimedia.org/wiki/File:Serenoa_repens_001.JPG

Schizandra: Photography by NoahElhardt May 13, 2006, under Public Domain.
http://commons.wikimedia.org/wiki/File:Drosera_schizandra_ne.jpg

Scullcap: Photography by USDA and Hafliger July 31, 2008, under Public Domain.
http://commons.wikimedia.org/wiki/File:Scutellaria_lateriflora.jpg

Shepherd's Purse: Photography by H. Zell May 2, 2009, under the terms of the GNU Free Documentation License, and the Creative Commons Attribution-Share Alike 3.0 Unported license.
http://commons.wikimedia.org/wiki/File:Capsella_bursa-pastoris_002.JPG

Slippery Elm: Photography by Phyzome March 20, 2005, under the terms of the GNU Free Documentation License, and the Creative Commons Attribution-Share Alike 3.0 Unported license.
http://commons.wikimedia.org/wiki/File:Ulmus_rubra_flowers.jpg

Solomon's Seal: Photography by Rasbak June 21, 2006, under the terms of the GNU Free Documentation License, and the Creative Commons Attribution-Share Alike 3.0 Unported license.
http://commons.wikimedia.org/wiki/File:Polygonatum_odoratum_resize.jpg

St. John's Wort: Photography by Aelwyn June 11, 2007, under the terms of the GNU Free Documentation License, and the Creative Commons Attribution-Share Alike 3.0 Unported license.
http://commons.wikimedia.org/wiki/File:Hypericum_perforatum_NRM.jpg

Tea Tree: Photography by Ethel Aardvark August 26, 2008, under the terms of the GNU Free Documentation License, and the Creative Commons Attribution-Share Alike 3.0 Unported license.
http://commons.wikimedia.org/wiki/File:Melaleuca_leucadendron_flowers.jpg

Thyme: Photography by H. Zell May 16, 2009, under the terms of the GNU Free Documentation License, and the Creative Commons Attribution-Share Alike 3.0 Unported license.
http://commons.wikimedia.org/wiki/File:Thymus_vulgaris_002.JPG

Turmeric: Photography by H. Zell November 15, 2009, under the terms of the GNU Free Documentation License, and the Creative Commons Attribution-Share Alike 3.0 Unported license.
http://commons.wikimedia.org/wiki/File:Curcuma_longa_001.JPG

Valerian: Photography by Pethan Utrecht June 19, 2005, under the terms of the GNU Free Documentation License, and the Creative Commons Attribution-Share Alike 3.0 Unported license.
http://commons.wikimedia.org/wiki/File:Valeriana_officinalis02.JPG

Violet: Photography by TeunSpaans March 31, 2005, under the terms of the GNU Free Documentation License, and the Creative Commons Attribution-Share Alike 3.0 Unported license.
http://commons.wikimedia.org/wiki/File:Viola-odorata-closeup.jpg

White Oak: Photography by Harborsparrow September 6, 2007, under Public Domain.
http://commons.wikimedia.org/wiki/File:Quercus_alba_leaf_spring.jpg

White Willow: Photography by Willow September 22, 2007 under the terms of the GNU Free Documentation License, and the Creative Commons Attribution-Share Alike 3.0 Unported license.
http://commons.wikimedia.org/wiki/File:Salix_alba_022.jpg

Witch Hazel: Photography by H. Zell December 9, 2009, under the terms of the GNU Free Documentation License, and the Creative Commons Attribution-Share Alike 3.0 Unported license.
http://commons.wikimedia.org/wiki/File:Hamamelis_virginiana_03.JPG

Wormwood: H. Zell July 29, 2009, under the terms of the GNU Free Documentation License, and the Creative Commons Attribution-Share Alike 3.0 Unported license.
http://commons.wikimedia.org/wiki/File:Artemisia_absinthium_0002.JPG

Yarrow: Photography by Pethan November 16, 2004, under the terms of the GNU Free Documentation License, and the Creative Commons Attribution-Share Alike 3.0 Unported license.
http://commons.wikimedia.org/wiki/File:Achillea_millefolium_bloem.jpg

Index

About the Author

I am a practicing herbalist of over twenty years. In practicing herbalism, I had become frustrated with having to cross-reference multiple resources in order to gather all of the necessary information on any one herb or disorder. It was time consuming and easily forgotten once the reason for the research had passed. Herbs for Life, which began fifteen years ago as my personal journal, takes all of this information from its various locations (books, nutritionists, herbalists, articles) and compiles it into a comprehensive and easy to follow book so that practitioners have everything they need in one location, formatted in a way that requires no extra research or legwork.

I learned herbalism from other herbalists and nutritionalists, books, and most anything I could lay my hands on. I have used this information to conduct panels and speeches at conventions, and to teach students interested in herbalism. I currently provide panels, lectures, and workshops on medicinal herbalism, essential oils, and other folklore or occult uses of herbs.

Website: www.kjdaoud.wordpress.com

Let us Capture your imagination!

CP

Captiva Press

Placida Publishing, LLC

www.placidapublishing.com
www.captivapress.com

CPSIA information can be obtained at www.ICGtesting.com
Printed in the USA
LVOW101023271011

252352LV00003B/3/P

9 781936 356171